P9-DFJ-709

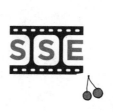

The Ultimate Guide To:

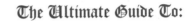

■ becoming a better flirt,

■ a tougher chick, and

■ a hotter girlfriend, and

■ to living life like a rock star

Carrie Borzillo-Vrenna

Cherry Bomb

SIMON SPOTLIGHT ENTERTAINMENT

New York London Toronto Sydney

Simon Spotlight Entertainment
A Division of Simon & Schuster, Inc.
1230 Avenue of the Americas
New York, NY 10020

Copyright © 2008 by Carrie Borzillo-Vrenna
Illustrations copyright © 2008 by Liz Adams

All rights reserved, including the right to reproduce this book or portions thereof in any form whatsoever. For information address Pocket Books Subsidiary Rights Department, 1230 Avenue of the Americas, New York, NY 10020.

First Simon Spotlight Entertainment hardcover edition August 2008

SIMON SPOTLIGHT ENTERTAINMENT and colophon are trademarks of Simon & Schuster, Inc.

For information about special discounts for bulk purchases, please contact Simon & Schuster Special Sales at 1-800-456-6798 or business@simonandschuster.com.

Interior design by Jaime Putorti

Manufactured in the United States of America

10 9 8 7 6 5 4 3 2 1

Library of Congress Cataloging-in-Publication Data

Borzillo-Vrenna, Carrie.
    Cherry bomb: the ultimate guide to becoming a better flirt, a tougher chick, and a hotter girlfriend, and to living life like a rock star / by Carrie Borzillo-Vrenna.—1st ed.
    p. cm.
    1. Women—Life skills guides.
    2. Women—Psychology. 3. Success. 4. Love. 5. Sex. 6. Wealth. I. Title.
    HQ1221.B77 2008
    646.70082—dc22

ISBN-13: 978-1-4169-6116-1
ISBN-10:   1-4169-6116-X

For chicks who rock

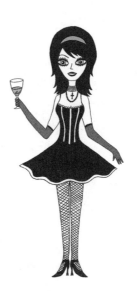

CONTENTS

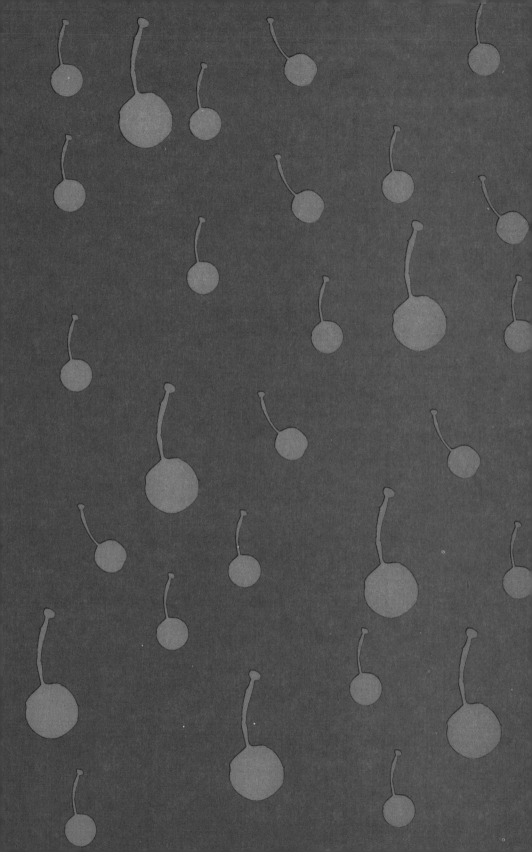

"Hello daddy, hello mom,
I'm your ch ch ch ch ch cherry bomb,
Hello world, I'm your wild girl,
I'm your ch ch ch ch ch cherry bomb."
~THE RUNAWAYS, "CHERRY BOMB"

INTRODUCTION

I've always been a little bit of a "wild girl," a rock chick, someone who is perfectly fine not fitting into the "girl next door" mold, who preferred playing "air band" with her friends as a young girl to donning a tutu and playing ballerina. Songs like "Cherry Bomb" by the Runaways—the 1960s/1970s teenaged girl group whose members were Joan Jett, Cherie Currie, Lita Ford, and Sandy West, who belted out rebellious songs while decked out in leather and lingerie—helped empower me with a tough and independent attitude and reinforced my inner badass.

I learned a lot from songs like this one and from songs by other strong females of the time. I learned to be defiant when necessary from Joan Jett & the Blackhearts'"Bad Reputation" ("A girl can do what she wants to do and that's what I'm gonna do!"). I learned to be "a real tough cookie" from Pat Benatar ("Hit Me with Your Best Shot"). And from a very young age I always walked into a party like I was walking onto a yacht (thank you "You're So Vain" by Carly Simon).

This strong, bold, edgy, musically obsessed, feisty mind-set is what inspired this book and what this book is all about. I wanted to write a new kind of girl-guide for women who don't always follow the rules, who prefer black nail polish to French manicures, who don't save the black fishnets just for Halloween, who wear Vivienne Westwood instead of Donna Karan, who prefer the bad boy, musician, or rebel over the jock, prep, or straightlaced businessman, and who live their lives (or at least aspire to) like a rock star.

This book is for the woman—the rock chick, if you will—who is not afraid to take chances, make a fool of herself, or boldly go for what she wants in life, be it a man, a better job, a new look, or a backstage pass. She is the girl who dares to be different, defiant, and oh so sexy and stylish while doing so. Rock chicks are not only female rock singers per se; they include women who embody a rebellious attitude, such as Joan of Arc, Frida Kahlo, Sandy at the end of *Grease*, Lara Croft, Leather Tuscadero, and countless others. A rock chick is a true maverick and a force to be reckoned with.

Cherry Bomb is essentially a lifestyle manual for rock chicks written by a rock chick, rock journalist, and rock wife. I've been a rock chick since age five, when I developed my first crush, on a dark-haired music man named Donny Osmond who had a penchant for wearing purple long before Prince did. By age seven, my music-loving parents had turned me on to the Beatles, the Rolling Stones, Queen, and David Bowie. By age eighteen, I had started my career as a music journalist writing for local fanzines back home in Connecticut.

Since then, I've written about the lives, styles, and relationships of rock stars and celebrities for music and entertainment magazines, including a stint as a sex and relationship advice columnist. As both a journalist and rock wife, I have clocked a lot of time backstage, on the road, at Hollywood parties, and entertaining friends and colleagues at home (who have dubbed me "Gotha Stewart" for my domestic—yet still rocking—skills on the party-throwing front).

All of my life, love, and career experiences have gone into *Cherry Bomb*. The advice, tips, and turn-ons in this book are things I've either done, lived, worn, used, witnessed, covered, tried, or been exposed to in one way or another. For a select few areas that I didn't have firsthand experience with when I started writing (like tying cherry stems in a knot with my tongue), I enlisted the help of friends, celebrities, designers, and experts to share their tips, advice, or words of inspiration.

There are some truly great girl-guides out there, but they are all for the modern girl, the bombshell, the fashionista, the single girl, the bad girl, the smart girl, the pinup, the vixen, or another specific type of girl. And while the rock chick I am, as well as the reader I have in mind for this book, might have a bit of all those personas in her, there hasn't been a guide written from a rock and roll point of view for women who rock their strong, confident, and sexy selves in an edgy, cool, and bold way. Until now.

Everyone has a little bit of rock chick in them—whether they know it yet or not. This book will help you embrace that wild side, or take your rock chick ways to the next level, or be turned onto some edgy cool stuff, or put a few new tricks up your sexy little sleeves. Or all of the above. I hope you enjoy reading *Cherry Bomb* as much as I enjoyed writing it for you.

~Carrie Borzillo-Vrenna
LOS ANGELES, JANUARY 2008

Joan Jett and Kim Fowley (the Runaways' cofounder, producer, and songwriter) wrote "Cherry Bomb" for me when I went in to audition for the Runaways. They wrote it right on the spot for me, and it was what they thought I was all about. I was fifteen, by the way. The "Cherry" part comes from my name, Cherie. I loved the song. I was a very rebellious girl at this point, and the words stuck real easy for me. I enjoyed singing it because it was the truth. "Cherry Bomb" is the epitome of what young girls feel when they go through a rebellious stage, which they all do. We all go through that stage where you don't want to listen to anyone and no one understands and you want to be independent and think you know it all. The line "hello world, I'm your wild girl" is basically about breaking out. When I was fifteen and singing that song in a corset, it empowered me. I think the song still empowers girls, young and old. It's like "Hey world, look at me. Look at what you created. Fuck you all." Even today, if a girl sings this song in front of her mirror, something will change in that girl.

~Cherie Currie of the Runaways
on "Cherry Bomb"

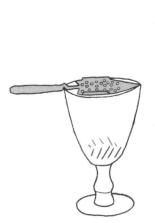

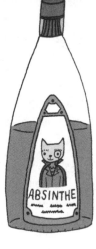

" Enough absinthe can crush
your spirit to the bone."
~BETH ORTON, "ABSINTHE"

ABSINTHE

Move over Jack Daniels. Absinthe is the new drink of choice for the rock and roll set. Marilyn Manson, Johnny Depp, Tommy Lee, OutKast, and Trent Reznor are among those who have enjoyed the intoxicant known as "The Green Fairy."

Why does absinthe rock? Much like the rock stars, artists, and celebrities who consume it, absinthe is the badass of all drinks, due to the legendary tales associated with it and with those who indulge in it. Absinthe's biggest claim to fame is that it's the substance blamed for Vincent van Gogh's cutting off his ear and sending it to his lover. Myth or fact? We'll never know.

So, what exactly is absinthe, you wonder? It's a green (and sometimes red) liqueur whose main ingredients are wormwood and anise. It tastes a bit like licorice. The feeling you get from it is best described as a combination of being alcohol-drunk and ecstasy-high. It kicks in fast, kicks in hard, and might lower your inhibitions more than even the strongest of whiskeys. Most drinkers will start feeling its magic midway through their first drink and describe the feeling as somewhat euphoric—warm, fuzzy, hazy, comfortable, relaxed, mellow, and oh so happy—yet they're surprisingly coherent and in-the-moment while in its grips.

CHERRY BOMB

Legendary writer Oscar Wilde once described being absinthe-drunk like this: "The first stage is like ordinary drinking, the second when you begin to see monstrous and cruel things. But if you can persevere you will enter in upon the third stage where you see things that you want to see."

Okay, before you get too excited, the absinthe you get today isn't quite as potent as the sometimes-lethal absinthe that Wilde, van Gogh, Ernest Hemingway, Pablo Picasso, and Edgar Allan Poe partied on way back when. But today's version does have a very high alcohol content—most new brands are between 65 and 70 percent, which is enough to make you forget portions of your night.

READY FOR YOUR NIGHT OF ABSINTHE? HERE'S WHAT YOU'LL NEED

YOUR SHOPPING LIST

■ A BOTTLE OF ABSINTHE: My favorite brands are Marilyn Manson's own Mansinthe and Red Serpis (both from www.absinthevertrieb.de), as well as Sebor (www.seborabsinth.com).

■ ABSINTHE GLASSES: The traditional glasses are a clear, cut glass in an egg shape or with a reservoir at the bottom. It's easy to find authentic 1890s French glasses at antique stores or online. The cuts in the glass indicate the "dose" of absinthe that should be poured.

■ ABSINTHE SAUCERS: In Paris cafés in the 1800s, the saucers would be marked with the prices of the drink.

■ ABSINTHE SPOON: A silver, perforated spoon with a ridge cut into it so it rests perfectly on the rim of an authentic absinthe glass. The diamond-shaped spoons were popular in the Belle Époque era.

■ SUGAR CUBES: You can get cubes at the grocery store or check out www.alandia.de to buy sugar cubes wrapped in black and green from World of Absinthe. You can buy glasses, spoons, and other absinthe accessories there too.

■ WATER: The colder the better.

■ FIRE: A lighter will do.

THE TRADITIONAL FRENCH RITUAL

STEP 1: Pour two shots of absinthe into a glass.

STEP 2: Rest the absinthe spoon on top of the glass.

STEP 3: Place one or two sugar cubes (to taste) on top of the spoon.

STEP 4: Pour another shot of absinthe over the sugar, soaking the cubes with the liqueur.

STEP 5: Light the absinthe-soaked sugar on fire and let the sugar burn until it caramelizes and starts melting into the glass. Be careful here: The blue flame is sometimes hard to see. Don't stick your finger in it to see if it's on fire—it is!

STEP 6: Pour a shot of ice-cold water over the fired-up sugar to put the fire out.

STEP 7: Stir any sugar that remains on the spoon into your absinthe. Once the water and sugar are stirred in, the Absinthe will "louche," which means to turn a milky white-green shade. And it's time to drink!

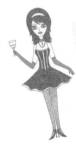

𝕲𝖔𝖙𝖍𝖆 𝕾𝖙𝖊𝖜𝖆𝖗𝖙 𝕿𝖎𝖕: *If that first sip sends shivers down your spine, and not in a good way, add more cold water and a little more sugar to sweeten it up. And don't forget—you won't taste a thing after you finish that first glass anyway!*

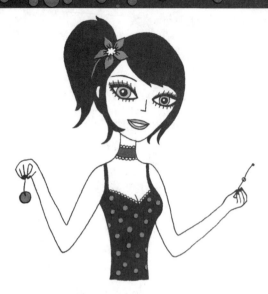

APPLE MARTINIS
AND THE CHERRY STEM TRICK

M ove over, mixologists! Cocktailing doesn't have to be as difficult as some recipes make it out to be. Forget about the fancy shakers, strainers, or jiggers. Here's a very simple way to make a very cool cocktail that is sure to impress:

STEP 1: Before serving, chill your martini glass (preferably a classic V-shaped clear martini glass) in the freezer.

STEP 2: After about ninety minutes of chilling, take your glass out of the freezer and pour in an equal amount of your favorite vodka (Grey Goose and Blavod rock!) and a green apple liqueur (like DeKuypers).

STEP 3: Stir with your finger, and be sure to lick off the excess seductively from your finger while staring at your object of affection.

STEP 4: Garnish with a maraschino cherry—stem on. You can use the naughty-looking nibbly bit to flirt with a cute guy. (Bonus points if you can tie that cherry stem into a knot!)

STEP 5: Add a very tiny splash of juice from the jar of cherries to the drink. But don't stir the cherry juice in (it'll turn an icky yellowish brown if you stir).

STEP 6: Assign a designated driver. This is a strong drink!

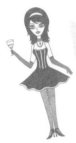

𝕲𝖔𝖙𝖍𝖆 𝕾𝖙𝖊𝖜𝖆𝖗𝖙 𝕿𝖎𝖕: *To get a frosty chill on the glass, rinse the glass in cold water, shake the excess water off so you don't have any large drops, then place the glass in the freezer until serving.*

HOW TO TIE A CHERRY STEM INTO A KNOT
(OTHERWISE KNOWN AS THE SUREFIRE WAY TO TURN ON THE GUY OF YOUR DREAMS!)

STEP 1: Seductively pull the juicy cherry off its stem, chew slowly, and swallow. Depending on how well you do the rest of the steps, this might be your sexiest move of this trick. So make it good.

STEP 2: Visualize a simple knot.

STEP 3: Have a friend ready with a camera.

STEP 4: Chew on the stem to soften it up a bit. But make sure you don't bite through the stem and cut it in half.

STEP 5: Using your tongue, fold the stem in half in your mouth.

STEP 6: Once folded, cross one of the ends slightly over the other.

STEP 7: Use your teeth to hold onto the crossed end while you use your tongue to move the other end through the loop.

STEP 8: Bite down on the crossed end and pull the other end with your tongue to tighten it up.

STEP 9: Don't lose the knot while you pull the stem out. Carefully, take it out of your mouth with your fingers.

STEP 10: Now, work it, girl! Show off this sucker to everyone in the bar and post a photo of it on your MySpace page. (Or post a video of you performing the trick on YouTube! That way no one will doubt your skills.)

> *We are shaped by our thoughts;*
> *we become what we think."*
>
> ~BUDDHA

ATTITUDE

No one rocked the ever-elusive internal confidence and peace more than Buddha did. "We become what we think." *Think* that you are awesome, and you shall become awesome. Think that you rock, and you too shall rock. Sure, Buddha probably didn't have rock in mind when he came up with that quote, but it certainly jives with today's "Fake it 'til you make it" or "If you think it, it will come" mind-set. And it works, whether you're going after a job, a new look, or the man of your dreams.

It also works in terms of sex appeal—if you feel sexy, others will think you are. We all know that true sex appeal has hardly anything to do with a perfectly symmetrical face, high cheekbones, ice blue eyes, or that 34-24-34 impossible-to-achieve figure. Sex appeal is all about being confident, feeling sensual, being comfortable in your own skin—whether you are a size 2 or a size 22—and having passion in your soul. If you think you are sexy, you will act sexy, and others will look at you as a sexy being.

Once your attitude is tuned into this, anything is possible.

CHERRY BOMB

11

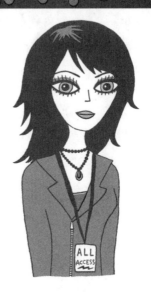

HOW TO GET BACKSTAGE
(WITHOUT BEING A WHORE!)

Sneaking backstage at a concert isn't as hard as it sounds. Nothing, really, is as hard as it sounds if you just rock it with confidence and style and use what you have. Being hot will only get you part of the way; the rest is all about using your noggin. This is how you do it:

FAN UP: Join the band's fan club on their official website and check for any offers to fan club members to go to a meet-and-greet. Or tune in to the local radio station or check the station's website for any contests to win backstage passes. I know, I know. It's not the coolest route, but it could get you to your destination.

SUCK UP TO THE HELP: By "help," I mean the opening band. Most times these newcomers don't have roadies to schlep their gear around. Show up early, offer to help unload their equipment, and ask for backstage passes. Or take your shot at them when they come offstage. If it's a small enough venue, the opening band might be out front watching the headliners along with the rest of the crowd. Go up to them and tell them you loved their show and ask if they have a pass to spare. Don't expect something for nothing—offer to buy them a drink or give them a puff off of your, er, cigarette.

If those methods don't work, there are other ways to get to the Promised Land that is backstage. Here they are:

SNEAKY WAY NO. 1: Walk in with an entourage of people who have passes. Pull the "I'm with them" move and waltz on by. The best way to waltz on by in any situation is to walk fast, talk on your cell as you're walking, and have that look on your face like you know where you're going, you belong there, and you'll bite someone's head off if they bother you.

SNEAKY WAY NO. 2: Get to the venue late morning/early afternoon before security is even there and when the crew is loading the equipment. Stow away in a bathroom (don't forget your hand sanitizer) and wait until the band shows up. For a 9 p.m. show the band could be getting cozy in their dressing rooms as early as 4 p.m., so that would be the time to come out of hiding in the bathroom and just "accidentally" walk by the dressing rooms. Hopefully, all will go well and you get to meet the band, tell them you think they rock, and ask them for an after-show pass. They might just be impressed with your backstage bravery enough to reward you with something sticky—and by that I mean a sticky pass! (See page 14.) But be prepared to get yelled at, kicked out, and embarrassed. Some bands and their crew will be cool; others won't.

SNEAKY WAY NO. 3: Get to the venue early, as in No. 2. Instead of stowing away near the toilets, make nice with the crew who are loading the equipment in and setting up the stage. But, ladies, no band is worth whoring yourself out for. So be nice to the staff but not THAT nice. If you're cool enough and not too stalker-ish, you might be able to befriend some of the crew guys at load-in and just ask for passes from them. For big festival shows, load-in can be as early as 7 a.m., so get to those shows early! Anyway, once you've become buddies with the friendly crew guy, ask him for passes or ask if he can walk you in.

SNEAKY WAY NO. 4: Get creative. A fan of pop-punk band New Found

CHERRY BOMB

Glory once dressed up in his pizza delivery outfit from work and just walked backstage saying he was delivering pizzas for the band. The fan met the band, but the guys weren't too thrilled when they discovered those pizza boxes he was holding were empty. So, if you go this route, make sure there is a hot and spicy pizza in the box. It sounds like something out of a bad teen movie, but it's a true story.

SNEAKY WAY NO. 5: I'll illustrate this one with an anecdote. Two friends of mine—authors of *How to Lose a Guy in 10 Days* Jeannie Long and Michele Alexander—showed up at the record release party for the band Orgy. They had walkie-talkies because, you know, club staff always have those Secret Service–like devices for their oh-so-important job of keeping people out. Plus they thought it would be fun to go out talking to each other on walkie-talkies. They were very official looking, and the ruse started out innocent enough. When they got to the party, they started to use their new toys to their advantage. They worked those walkie-talkies like pros, marched right up to the front of the line, and voila! the velvet rope was instantly opened and they scurried right in. Once inside, they were able to go into the stairwells, backstage, and other areas the general public couldn't go to because everyone thought they worked there. Enough said.

$\mathfrak{P}$ASS HIERARCHY

So, you got the pass. Now what? You need to know just what that pass means. Here's the lowdown on backstage passes, from the least amount of access to the most:

"AFTER-SHOW" STICKY PASS: This is the pass that crews often give to pretty girls they think are easy—the passes that just about anyone can get. They might get you past the security guard, but you usually end up in a "holding pen," where the artist may or may not make an appearance after the show. Regardless, you are technically "backstage." Yeah, you!

"GUEST" STICKY PASS: Whoever gave you this pass, cling to their side like there's no tomorrow. You are their guest. And if they are a good host, they will introduce you to someone in the band. Or at least get you a free beer from a dressing room.

"WORKING" STICKY PASS: This one takes a bit of faking it. It's a pass reserved for people who are working the show in some capacity. You clearly are not, so try not to get caught. Don't make eye contact with anyone, and act low-key. It should get you far enough to pass the drummer in the hallway at least. Be prepared to get kicked out on your ass if security or anyone else in authority finds out.

"V.I.P." LAMINATED PASS: You're in like Flynn with this one. You can go anywhere, but you shouldn't. See Dos and Don'ts below to avoid any backstage faux pas.

"ALL ACCESS" LAMINATED PASS: This one's reserved for wives, girlfriends, family members, mangers, agents, and label reps of the band. If you are none of the above and you got this pass, it means someone thinks they are scoring with you tonight. Careful here.

BACKSTAGE DOS AND DON'TS

DO: Be polite. Tell the band that you enjoyed the show.
DON'T: Gush about their performance or critique it. They don't need to know that you thought the guitar solo was too long or that someone was out of tune on song number two.

DO: Be interesting, fun, and charming.
DON'T: Try to be the center of attention.

DO: Act like you belong—be cool, laid back.
DON'T: Look mega-stars like Prince, Beyoncé, or Mariah Carey in the eyes. Ever.

DO: Think about what you want to say before you meet the band members.
DON'T: Get stumped after your first "hello."

DO: Dress rock and roll cool.

DON'T: Wear the band's merchandise that they sell at the show backstage or dress like a groupie. (See page 177 for some style help.)

DO: Be respectful.

DON'T: Walk into a dressing room, tour bus, or "artist only" area without an escort.

DO: Mind your table manners.

DON'T: Grab food and drinks on your own. Wait for someone to offer them to you. And never take the last of anything—the last bottle of water, beer, or even the last piece of sweaty cheese on the deli platter.

DO: Be quick. Have a goal. Reach it. Get out.

DON'T: Overstay your welcome or whine if security asks you to leave.

DO: Bring a camera, make sure your lips are glossed, and be ready to strike a pose with your favorite band member.

DON'T: Take a pic without asking permission first. You are not the paparazzi!

BITCHY BROADS

*L*et's face it—women can be brutal to one another. But the first thing you must understand when a broad is bitchy to you is that there are usually three main reasons for her bitchiness:

1 You did something to deserve it, and if so, that's your own fault, so deal with it.

2 She is jealous of you, of your man, of your job, or how others like you better than her.

3 She is insecure and only feels better when making others feel like shit.

Usually, it's no. 2 or 3, and if you're an empathetic person, you might actually feel sad for her deep level of self-hate. But screw that! It's time to put the bitch in her place. At this point there is no need to waste any more mental energy on figuring her out. You need to examine the situations and figure out how to come out on top. Here are three examples of bitches and how to ward them off:

CHERRY BOMB

17

THE PATRONIZER: The woman who gets off on the misfortune of others and tries to make herself feel better by using backhanded sympathy or commiseration.

She Says: "I'm so sorry to hear that Erik dumped you! I actually saw him last night at the Roxy making out with some woman, but she wasn't nearly as pretty as you."

You Say: "That's nice. Hey, do you have any quarters? I need to put money in the meter." Then you walk away and tell one of your real friends what a loser that bitch is.

Why? You don't ever want to let the Patronizer know she's gotten to you, because she'll just keep twisting the proverbial knife deeper every time she has an opportunity to get a rise out of you. Of course you probably are upset, but if you avoid engaging her, eventually she'll just move on to someone who's not as strong as you.

THE CONDESCENDER: The woman who masks an insult as a compliment in an effort to TRY to make you doubt yourself or feel bad.

She Says: "Those pants make you look skinny. Are they that stretch corduroy?"

You Say: "Yes, actually they are. You should get a pair. You'd look skinny in them too!"

Why? The Condescender loves to see a hurt look on someone's face when she's delivered one of her nasty-nice compliments—it makes her feel superior. Don't fall for it!

THE ALIENATOR: She loves to put you on the spot by making an uncalled-for or embarrassing remark about you right in front of a new boyfriend or a group that doesn't know you that well.

She Says: "You used to be such a party girl—remember the time you were giving [insert name of rock star] a blow job and you puked all over him because you had ten Jack and Cokes?"

You Say: "Was it only ten?"

Why? The Alienator is a sadist. And while she is completely insecure, she's also a control freak who gets off on humiliating people. But if you don't feel humiliated, then she failed. So just let it roll off of you.

BOTTLE SERVICE

ottle service is a way to buy VIP status at the hottest night-clubs. It's a way to feel like a rock star for a night. And, more important, bottle service pretty much guarantees a hassle-free night out at the city's hardest-to-get-into clubs. So, what is bottle service exactly? It's when a nightclub, bar, or lounge allows patrons to buy a full bottle of booze instead of paying for drinks one at a time. With that you get to skip the line to get into the club and your own private table. Sounds pretty simple, eh? Well, it's not quite as easy as it seems. Though it varies from club to club and city to city, here's a basic rundown of how it works and what you need to know:

BEFORE YOU BOOK IT: Work your connections to try to get on the guest list and get a table for free, or pal up with a better-connected friend and attach yourself to his or her table. Don't have friends in high places? Read on.

DO YOUR HOMEWORK: Not every club offers the same amount of hospitality with their bottle service. Research the clubs online or call them up and ask how their bottle service works. What you're looking for is this: With your reservation for a table and a bottle, you and your pals should get free admission to the club, not have to wait in line to get in, have your own private table with a waitress, and get your mixers (OJ, cranberry, tonic, and club soda are the norm; Red Bull will cost a little extra), ice, and garnishes for your drinks for free. You can even get free refills on the mixers.

Make reservations as far in advance as possible. Ask what the minimum is—it's usually one bottle per four free passes. Don't expect to have a table of eight people and just order one bottle. That ain't gonna happen. Ask about extra services too. For instance, at club Area in L.A., they offer a Tableside Mixology Program so you don't have to mix your own drinks.

LOAD UP ON THE CASH: This service is not for people with shallow pockets. It will run a pretty penny, but you can shave a few dimes off the cost if you do a little comparison shopping. Like I said, not every club is the same, so if you don't have your heart set on a specific club, shop around a bit. An average bottle of vodka in most cities runs between $250 and $300. At LAX in Los Angeles on a Thursday night, we're talking $325 for a bottle of Belvedere; $375 for Grey Goose. But at Privilege in L.A., Grey Goose is $25 cheaper at $350 a bottle, and they also offer up the way-cheaper Effen (pronounced F-ing) for just $290. Also beware that a 20% tip is usually added to your bill or expected. No 12% tipping here, folks. Not cool.

ADD IT UP: If you're still thinking it seems insane to part with this kind of cash, let me break it down for you. If you and your three pals wanted to go to the hottest club in town without bottle service, you could be paying $20 a pop to get in. That's $80 in cover charges. In L.A., the average drink costs between $11 and $15. Let's call it $13 a drink. If you guys are truly partying like rock stars, you're gonna be drinking at least four drinks each. That's $208 (not including tip) on drinks for your party. We're at $288 now. Subtract that from a $325 bottle of vodka, and your party of four is only paying $37 more for bottle service. That turns out to just $9.25 per person, and for that extra $9.25 each you get your own exclusive table, you don't have to wait in line at the door or at the bar, and you feel pretty darn special in the process. Totally worth it!

Note: Bottle service normally means a 750 ml bottle, which is 25.35 ounces. If you pour 1.5 ounces for each drink, you get 16.9 drinks from that bottle, which averages 4.25 drinks each.

BUDDY UP, BITCHES! Bottle service is really worth it when you're rolling with four people who all want to drink the same thing. Pick your buddies wisely; agree on which libation you all want to drink ahead of time and decide whose credit card it's going down on. Most clubs don't like splitting things four ways, so work it out among yourselves before you go.

WHY IT ROCKS: You know the dread you feel when you roll up to a club and see a long line at the door and a scowling doorman with a clipboard shaking his head "no" a lot? Yeah, well, when you opt for a night out with bottle service, that scenario doesn't exist for you. Instead, when you roll up to the man with the clipboard, you can confidently give him your name, he unhooks that velvet rope for you, and you waltz right in. You might even be seated at a table next to your favorite rock star. Bonus perk: Some clubs let other patrons occupy your table until you show up. So, once you show up, you have the pleasure of kicking those people out of your VIP area. Last but not least, going the bottle service route also means that you can safely wear those sky-high stilettos, because you'll have your own cozy, private place to rest those feet between dancing and trolling for guys.

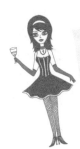

𝕲𝖔𝖙𝖍𝖆 𝕾𝖙𝖊𝖜𝖆𝖗𝖙 𝕿𝖎𝖕: *One of the best bottle service deals in Los Angeles is the $150 bottle of Veuve Clicquot (yellow label) at the world famous Viper Room.*

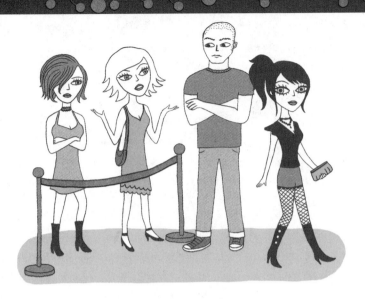

BOUNCERS

If you don't go the bottle service route and you're not on a guest list (see page 91 so you won't make that mistake again!), then you will have to deal with an (oftentimes bitchy) bouncer. Melissa Renee Hernandez and Anna Geyer, co-talent buyer and marketing coordinator, respectively, at the Viper Room in L.A., give us the skinny on how to best act when your plan is to just walk up to the club and hope to get in:

If you're a pretty girl and you go to the front of the line, if it's late enough, the door guy will probably let you in. But you can't just be a pretty girl and stand there and expect the velvet rope to drop. You need to say something like, "Hey, can I come in? How long is the wait?" Have a goal and be aggressive, but not too aggressive. Don't be rude and don't pull an attitude by saying something like, "Don't you know who I am?" You'll just look like an asshole. Don't argue. Be patient. Bouncers don't have to be nice. It's not in their job requirement to be sweet, so don't expect that from them or be shocked or upset if they are snippy with you. Some guys grease their palms, and that can work too. If you show up with a business card and you work someplace cool, flash your card, and if the doorman is nice, he'll probably let you in, though Casper, our doorman, might just say, "What? Do you need me to recycle this for you?"

BREAKUP SONGS

Nothing helps mend a broken heart like rocking out to some "I hate you!" song by a woman who never lets a man get her down. Followed, of course, by wallowing while listening to self-pity songs and eating a pint of ice cream. But to fully mourn the loss of a relationship, one needs to move through the five stages of grief, a concept Swiss psychiatrist Elisabeth Kübler-Ross introduced in her 1969 book, *On Death and Dying*. And I've got the perfect song for each stage to help you work through your heartbreak.

FIVE STAGES OF GRIEF PLAYLIST

STAGE 1: Denial; Sheryl Crow, "It Don't Hurt"

STAGE 2: Anger; Alanis Morissette, "You Oughta Know"

STAGE 3: Bargaining; The Cardigans, "Lovefool"

STAGE 4: Depression; Amy Winehouse, "Love Is a Losing Game"

STAGE 5: Acceptance; Gloria Gaynor, "I Will Survive"

CHERRY BOMB

Since most of us spend a lot of time in the Anger and Depression stages, I've compiled an expanded set list for those trying times:

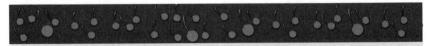

Songs to Vacuum Fast To
(aka the Anger stage)

Carrie Underwood, "Before He Cheats"
Nancy Sinatra, "These Boots Are Made for Walkin'"
Pat Benatar, "Heartbreaker"
Kim Wilde, "You Keep Me Hangin' On"
No Doubt, "Happy Now?"
Melissa Etheridge, "Bring Me Some Water"
Janis Joplin, "Piece of My Heart"
The Murmurs, "You Suck"
Scandal, "Goodbye to You"
Drill, "Go to Hell"
Kelis, "Caught Out There"
Lush, "Ciao!"

Songs to Eat a Pint of Ice Cream To
(aka the Depression stage)

Yeah Yeah Yeahs, "Maps"
Patsy Cline, "Crazy"
No Doubt, "Don't Speak"
Carole King, "It's Too Late"
Olivia Newton-John, "Hopelessly Devoted to You"
Toni Braxton, "Un-Break My Heart"
Billie Holiday, "I'm a Fool to Want You"
The Supremes, "Where Did Our Love Go?"
Lisa Loeb, "Stay (I Missed You)"

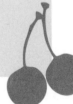

BREAST CANCER AWARENESS

By fashion designer and breast cancer survivor Betsey Johnson

"My breast implants had deflated, so I had them taken out. About three or four days after that surgery, I was in bed in my country house laying on my back, and I was feeling around to check out the scars and how they were healing. I had the little half-inch cut where they had taken the implants out, and I could tell what was scar tissue near the cut, but then there was a little thing on the left side. My doctors and I found out it was a little tumor, just ten milligrams. We got it right away with radiation. The key thing is that you just have to lie on your back and feel around and not be afraid to call your doctor if you feel something that doesn't seem right. I know it's a weird thing because you don't want to discover anything bad, but it is really crucial to check yourself. If you have breast cancer in your family, you should get checked as early as age twelve. I'd had a mammogram six months before I discovered the lump and it had come out negative, so it's important to check regularly. Mammograms and sonograms are crucial because it's all about early detection.

CHERRY BOMB

BRITISH BLOKES

(Or How to attract, seduce, and understand a bloke from Blighty)

There's a reason why Madonna, Gwen Stefani, Gwyneth Paltrow, and Liv Tyler have all married creative creatures from Britain: (a) British men are just so chivalrous; (b) okay, the accent doesn't hurt either.

But before an American woman can saddle up to a Brit, there are a few things she needs to know about his dating practices and slang. For this exercise, I enlisted the help of my British gal pal Nicole Powers, who is married to British rock star Leigh Gorman, of Bow Wow Wow fame. Here is what she had to say:

The way to flirt with a British man is not by flirting but by talking about football or British TV and drinking a LOT of beer. Aggressive American-style flirting would just put the fear of God into a Brit boy and would likely have the opposite effect as the one desired. They are just too socially awkward and easily embarrassed for that kind of behavior.

An opening line such as "Can you explain the offside rule?" will likely be more successful than the lame "Do you come here often?" or "I like your accent!" And don't even pull the "act stupid to flirt" MO by giggling over the whole football/soccer thing. They take their "football" seriously. Yes, football to the Brits is soccer to Americans. Get over it. Another good conversation-starter could involve anything on *Doctor Who*. While most of the world debates which James Bond film is the best, hip Brits are more interested in which *Doctor Who* is the definitive one.

You will also need a sharp wit, as British pub conversation is practically a competitive sport. Getting your wit on is the best way to get noticed. She who jokes best wins the respect of her peers, as well as his heart. Once you've struck up a good conversation, relax and let the beer take care of the rest. Speaking of beer, the mating ritual of a British bloke generally involves him getting rat-arsed (very, very drunk) with a potential prospect before "copping off" (disappearing for some sexual interaction) with her at a point when all inhibitions have disappeared along with the beer. If you're lucky, he'll be drunk enough to ask for your number yet sober enough to remember it, which means you're well on your way to taking the relationship to the next level.

Don't expect any properly planned out "dates" with your Brit boy. First, they don't use the word *dating*. It's simply "going out" to them. And, second, instead of making a big to-do of "going out" with you, they may just simply arrange to be in the vicinity of you and a pint of beer at a future point by asking if you fancy going out somewhere at some predetermined time. Indeed, you may only be certain whether such an appointment is a date after the fact, and even then it's not always clear, but that just goes with the territory when dating a Brit.

ENGLISH-TO-ENGLISH DICTIONARY

If you don't know the British meaning of some of these words, you might end up slapping the poor bloke across the face, having a bad "lost in translation" moment, or making a fool of yourself if he says,

CHERRY BOMB

"I'm pissed!" and you reply, "Why? What's wrong?" Read on for a quick English-to-English primer:

FOOTBALL

American meaning: A sport played by 300-pound men in helmets and spandex who try to move a pigskin ball to the end of the field with their hands.

British meaning: A sport played by model-esque pretty boys like David Beckham where they try to move a round ball to the end of the "pitch" with their feet (aka soccer).

SHAG

American meaning: A cute, choppy, layered haircut.
British meaning: To have sex.

PISSED

American meaning: Mad, angry.
British meaning: Drunk.

BIRD

American meaning: A flying feathery thing. Or to raise your middle finger to say "fuck you," as in "to give the bird."
British meaning: A girl.

CELEBRITY PICKUP TIPS

ou've already learned how to not come off as a crazed groupie when you meet someone famous, so now it's time to put your newfound skills into action. In addition to sneaking backstage, there are plenty of places to meet this A-list crush of yours that don't involve camping outside the recording studio, following the tour bus on long drives, or pacing outside the movie set or TV studio. Instead, you want to be in a natural setting, like a park, restaurant, bar, coffee shop, or gas station. Or if you hit the jackpot and end up as an invited guest (or a pal's "plus one") at a Hollywood party, movie premiere, or charity event, even better!

Now that you've spotted your celebrity crush in a location or situation that won't have you pegged as a stalker, here's how you make your move:

SPILL A DRINK ON HIM! Works: Anywhere drinking is acceptable. Okay, I know this sounds like an awful thing to do, but it worked for Calista Flockhart. She spilled a drink on Harrison Ford at the 2002 Golden Globe Awards and they've been blissed out in love ever since. But be kind—make sure the drink is clear and that your glass is only a quarter

CHERRY BOMB

full. You don't want to soak and stain the guy's super-expensive Galliano suit. Be cute in your apology. Take your napkin and start to wipe off your spilled drink—if it's on his crotch, don't be shy! He's bound to politely brush your hand away and let you off the hook. Look him in the eyes with your sexiest doe-eyed expression and ask, "Can I make it up to you by buying you a drink? I promise I won't spill this one." That is some kick-ass foreplay to a guy who is interested.

USE YOUR DOG! Works: At a dog park, duh. If the celeb is a true animal lover, he'll be out at the dog park with the pooper-scooper himself instead of having his assistant do his dirty work. (Those living in Los Angeles should make a beeline to the celeb-filled Laurel Canyon Dog Park.) When he's not looking, throw your dog's toy in the direction of the celeb's dog, and if all goes well, you'll be making small flirty talk with the hunky celeb in no time. If you get so lucky as to pet the celeb's dog and you and the furry one hit it off, you can say something cheeky like, "Your dog has good taste in women." Or if the pups aren't playful, just sit on the bench next to him and ignore him. If you're his type, he'll start talking to you, and he'll likely be intrigued by your lack of interest. Being indifferent has its appeal.

GET SASSY: Works: Anywhere. If you're standing behind him, you can mumble, "Nice butt" and giggle a bit. Or if you're standing with a girlfriend, whisper to her, "He's so hot." His ego will surely make him turn around to see who paid him the compliment. When he does, act embarrassed and then say, "Well, it's true. You *do* have a nice butt." If he's interested, he'll take it from there. Josh Duhamel used a similar approach on Fergie. The pair met when Fergie guest-starred on his TV show, *Las Vegas*. His opening line to her was "You're hot."

PLAY DUMB: Works: Anywhere except on the set of his movie/TV show, at the premiere of his latest film, or at his band's show. Let's say that you've struck up a conversation with your celeb crush and it's gotten to the point when you should introduce yourselves. He's likely going to assume that you know who he is. But you need to pretend like you haven't a clue. Ask him for his name. If he says his first and last name, say, "Oh. [Giggle] I didn't recognize you. I just thought you were some cute guy." If he only says his first name, then ask him what he does. Maybe say something sassy like, "Let me guess, you're a model." When he says he's in a band or he's an actor, look up, giggle, and say, "Oh, sorry." He'll probably be pleasantly surprised that you didn't instantly recognize him. And he'll be happy to know right off the bat that you aren't his "number one fan." Of course, don't be foolish here. This scenario won't be believable if the celeb in question is hugely famous, like a Johnny Depp type, but chances of a star of that caliber being in a natural setting chatting up a stranger are pretty slim.

If any of these situations go well and the two of you are flirting and vibing, then before you leave, hand him your card and tell him you'd like to grab a drink sometime, then say good-bye and walk away. This means you need to have your card ready to go—put it in your back pocket or in the outer flap of your bag. You don't want to search for paper and a pen or even fumble for the card, especially if he didn't even ask for your number. You also don't want to linger long enough for him to feel obligated to reciprocate. Do it fast and with a smile—"Here's my card. Call me if you want." Walk away. Nice and clean. If you don't have a job that requires having a business card, have some made. You can get them for free at vistaprint.com. Print some up featuring your name, phone number, and email address (it doesn't have to say what you do). Do not put your home address on it—that's just not safe!

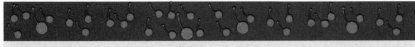

Don'ts!

- Don't gush about his latest album, movie, or play.
- Don't stalk him.
- Don't be pushy, sleazy, or overzealous.
- Don't quote lyrics from his song or dialogue from his movie.
- If it's going well, no matter what, you should never, ever, ever say, "You had me at hello."
- Don't overstay your welcome. If he's not flirty after the first few moments of meeting, cut your losses and walk away.
- Never, ever, ever, ever admit that you named a pet after him.

CHERRY BOMB

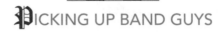

SINGER

Where to find him: Center of the room or holding court in the VIP section.

Characteristics: Self-centered, egomaniacal, selfish, and narcissistic on the inside, but cool, coy, and carefree on the outside. Tries to act aloof but ends up drawing more attention to himself in doing so.

How to hit on him: Be as chill and low-key as he's trying to be. Talk to him about his vintage car collection instead of his band.

GUITARIST

Where to find him: In the singer's shadow talking smack about him with a nemesis.

Characteristics: Outgoing, life of the party, attention seeking, prone to showboating, argumentative, competitive, the asshole of the bunch.

How to hit on him: Ignore the singer and lavish your affections on him instead. Stroke his ego, but don't overdo it.

BASSIST

Where to find him: At the bar or with a chick in the dressing room.

Characteristics: Moody, pissy, bitchy, always sulking or complaining. Classic middle child syndrome.

How to hit on him: Buy him a shot and join in on whatever he's bitching about. Misery loves company!

DRUMMER

Where to find him: He's the guy in the corner who no one is paying attention to; or he's the guy in the Rush T-shirt.

Characteristics: Lonely, plagued by an inferiority complex, left out of the fun and games, great biceps.

How to hit on him: Just talk to him and he's yours! Work in Neil Peart and you might just get a marriage proposal on the spot.

KEYBOARDIST

Where to find him: Deep in a serious conversation with someone about something important—history, politics, technology, or Bob Moog.

Characteristics: He's the smartest and nerdiest of all the band guys. He makes good use of both sides of his brain.

How to hit on him: Talk tech (ProTools vs. Logic) or discuss video games ("Halo 3" vs. "World of Warcraft").

PROS AND CONS OF DATING MUSICIANS

PROS	CONS
Devilishly sexy	Sexually promiscuous
Mysterious	Mischievous
Skinny	Skinnier than you
In touch with his emotions	Moody
Great hair	Mirror hog
Self-aware	Selfish
Godlike stage presence	Thinks he's God's gift to women
Makes you great mix CDs	Mixes up your name with another girl's
Gets you concert tickets	Gets to sleep until noon the next day while you scramble to make it to work by 9:30 a.m.
"Songwriter-sensitive"	Cries at every movie

CHROME HEARTS

What Makes Chrome Hearts Rock?

When you think of high-end Gothic rock and roll accessories, two words come to mind: Chrome Hearts.

The brand, founded by motorcycle enthusiast Richard Stark, is known for their chunky, expensive, and often-copied silver jewelry adorned with crosses, fleurs-de-lis, daggers, florals, Celtic motifs, and, of course, hearts. They're equally known for their leather pants and Goth furniture.

And, of course, nothing screams rock and roll rebel like a good old-fashioned "fuck you" does, so Chrome Hearts stamps that pleasantry on some of their tanks, tees, and even bath towels. (The store, tucked away on Robertson Blvd. in Los Angeles, even has a Fuck You welcome mat. But, unfortunately, it's not for sale.)

Chrome Hearts was once favored only by tougher rockers like Cher and Tommy Lee and their entourages, but they've become the brand that more mainstream celebrities such as Paris Hilton or Lindsay Lohan like to rock when they want to look edgier. Likewise, high-end conservative brands such as Rolex and Baccarat have teamed with the company to create edgier lines as well. (Case in point: Jessica Simpson bought a decked-out vintage Chrome Hearts-Rolex with diamonds for her sister Ashlee on her twenty-first birthday.)

But to sport some true rock and roll extravagance, one needs to look at the Chrome Hearts' myriad everyday housewares that bear their crosses. For instance, you can get a silver Chrome Hearts cap for your tube of toothpaste, as well as Chrome Hearts paper clips, scissors, staplers, doorknobs, drawer knobs, and more. In addition, you can take in your Levi's or a pair of sneakers and have Chrome Hearts "rock them up" for you by replacing the existing hardware with their silver studs or by adding leather cross patches.

If you're not ready to plop down a wad of green to make your toothpaste look cool or turn your $50 Levi's into a pair of $500 Chrome Hearts Levi's, then just spring for the Fuck You tank top, a cross-adorned skull cap, or their signature sunglasses to make your statement.

Oh, and don't let the name fool you. There's no chrome here. It's all silver, platinum, and gold.

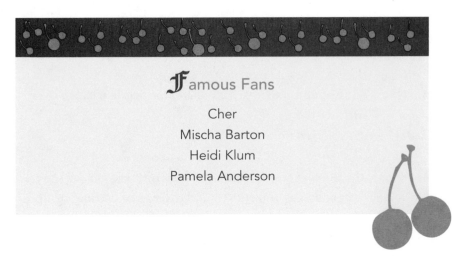

Famous Fans

Cher
Mischa Barton
Heidi Klum
Pamela Anderson

CLUBBING

A Quick A–Z Guide

Act cool.

Bouncers have the power to, well, bounce you outta the club. Be nice and polite to them.

Club vs. bar. Rockers like bars. Actors and models like clubs.

Dance with your girlfriends.

Exit gracefully. Don't stumble out of the club drunk, puking, or pulling a chick's hair, unless you don't mind a video of it showing up on *TMZ* or YouTube.

Frolic with friends you trust. Never go to a club alone or only with a frienemy. Nothing is worse than being left at a club because your "friend" ditched you for a dude.

Guest lists. Try to get on one. If you work in the industry at all, call the club promoter or rep and ask nicely.

Hide your stare under your hair. A well-tipped hat or glasses will also do when you don't want to get caught staring at a celeb or hottie from across the room.

Impress with your dress. Find out the dress code before going out and coordinate with pals. Nothing puts a damper on your time out if one of you is completely made up and the other is in jeans and flats.

Jerks. If a guy comes up to you and opens with "Hey, can you settle a bet for me and my friend . . ." or "Hey ladies, I need a female opinion on something . . ." run away. Those are the opening "lines" taught by goggles-loving pickup "artist" "Mystery."

Keep your drink where you can see it. Too many people get dosed with "date rape" drugs these days when they leave their drink at a table or bar counter near creepy men.

Let him know you're interested. Don't just stare at that cute guy; go ahead and make a move.

Munch! If the night's coming to an end and you're feeling a little too drunk to move, grab something to eat to sober up a bit. Even if it's just munching on nuts from the bar, it will help! (And nuts are healthier than that slice of pizza from the place around the corner when you exit the club.)

Never mix drinks. The old phrase "Liquor before beer, we're in the clear. Beer before liquor never sicker" isn't really true. Beer usually is okay with most other drinks—a shot and a beer, whiskey with a beer chaser, even beer and wine in the same night isn't going to leave you facedown in porcelain. White wine and champagne are usually okay to drink in one night too. But try any other combinations (especially wine and whiskey!) and you're in trouble!

CHERRY BOMB

Oh-no. You left your credit card at the club. Don't panic. It happens a lot. Call the club immediately after realizing your mistake. They are used to this and usually hold the card until the cardholder calls.

Prearranged designated drivers are your friends. If that fails, find another mode of transportation that doesn't involve your getting behind the wheel while intoxicated. And a cab, a subway, or even car service is cheaper than the price you would pay if you get a DUI.

Quickies. Every gal should have sex with her man at least once in a club bathroom or in a VIP booth that has curtains.

ROCKSTAR or Red Bull energy drinks are better and cheaper than drugs when you're planning on staying up all night partying.

Save money by drinking smart. Show up early for happy hour or choose wine or well liquor (well liquor is the house liquor, as in the cheapest available) over a more expensive mixed drink with top-shelf liquor.

Tipping. $1 per drink. $2–3 for valet. $1 per bathroom visit. $1–2 for coat check. 20% of bill for food. If you want stronger drinks or for the bartender to take care of you faster, tip at least $2 on your first drink.

Unthankful equals uncool. If you got on a guest list or were invited into someone else's VIP booth, don't forget your manners. Being un-thankful won't get you another invitation the next time you party at that club.

VIP booths. The best way to get a booth or table is to order bottle service in advance. Trust me, it's worth it.

Water. For every alcoholic drink you imbibe, drink one glass of water. Hydration helps prevent hangovers!

X Your ex walks into the club with a hot new girlfriend. Don't do what most chicks do and spy on him all night, act out in front of him in an attempt to show off, or make out with a loser to make him jealous. Just ignore him and have fun!

Yes! Why go to a pool hall, dance club, karaoke joint, or British pub with a great dart board if you're not going to partake in any of those activities? Just Say Yes to participating in whatever the venue has to offer, even if you totally blow at said activity.

Zero toleration for drunk drivers. If you designated a driver but she or he got drunk anyway, please steal the keys and call a cab. Forget about hurting yourself. Think about the puppy she might run over or the innocent mother of two she could mow down in a moment of bad judgment.

CONFIDENCE

"Always act like you're wearing an invisible crown."

~AUTHOR UNKNOWN

"I think I was born strong-willed. That's not the kind of thing you can learn. The advantage is you stick to what you believe in and rarely get pushed out of what you want to do."

~JOAN JETT

"Nobody can make you feel inferior without your consent."

~ELEANOR ROOSEVELT

"The best way to gain self-confidence is to do what you are afraid to do."

~AUTHOR UNKNOWN

"I was always looking outside myself for strength and confidence, but it comes from within. It is there all the time."

~PSYCHOTHERAPIST ANNA FREUD

DANCING TIPS

By Cheryl Burke of Dancing with the Stars

■ If someone asks you to dance, just do it, have fun, and try not to worry if you are a good dancer or not.

■ Keep it simple. Don't go all crazy with dance moves. The most basic move you should try to master is the simple step to the side, touch, side, touch, side, touch. While you're sidestepping, let your arms swing out naturally with your body.

■ Save the hand claps or finger snaps for when the song calls for them, but don't do them throughout the whole song.

■ Keep your eyes off the floor and on your dance partner, the cute guy across the room, or just on your surroundings in general.

■ Do not sing to the song you are dancing to! Smile, talk to your friends, but don't sing.

■ If you see someone with good moves on the dance floor, try to copy them a bit.

■ Remember, dancing isn't just fun, it's good for you! It's a great form of exercise, and you won't even notice that you are dancing off the pounds, because it's fun. Dancing also helps keep you sober when you are out partying with your friends, because when you dance, you sweat out the alcohol. It also makes you want to drink more water, so it keeps you hydrated.

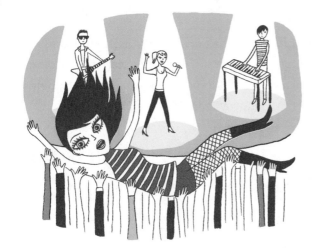

"Life shrinks or expands in proportion to one's courage."

~ANAÏS NIN,
DIARY, 1969

DARING DAMES

Forget the truth part of Truth or Dare. The dare part is so much more fun. But before you can dare others to do silly stuff, you need the courage to be a daring dame on your own. You don't get anywhere in life without breaking out of your shell a bit, expanding your boundaries, or even making a fool out of yourself. Try each of these fun and daring deeds at least once. You may discover a new you!

1 *Dare to be sexy:* Pole dance! Go to amateur night at the strip club or just use a street sign pole while you're waiting outside a club.

2 *Dare to be a rock star:* Sing Alanis Morissette's "You Oughta Know" or Nine Inch Nails'"Closer" (you know, the song that goes, "I want to f*&k you like an animal") at the top of your lungs in a cute boy's face at a karaoke bar.

3 *Dare to be flirty:* Pinch a stranger's butt and walk away.

4 *Dare to be dangerous:* Stage dive at a punk rock show.

CHERRY BOMB

5 *Dare to be forward:* Out of the blue, plant a kiss on the cute guy you're talking to.

6 *Dare to be racy:* Don't wear panties under your dress. But keep the legs closed when you exit the car. You want to be daring, not dumb. Blondie's Debbie Harry used to go commando with class long before twits like Britney, Paris, and Lindsay made it trashy.

> *People have speculated about whether I was wearing knickers when I appeared on stage in a really short dress, and there were occasions when I went out without underwear, but I'm not flashing myself like Britney. I don't think I ever went out on stage without some kind of underwear, because of the front row. God knows, though, I may have."*
>
> ~BLONDIE'S DEBBIE HARRY *(TIMES ONLINE U.K.)*

7 *Dare to be free:* Go to a nude beach.

8 *Dare to be irresponsible:* Spend your rent money on an amazing new party dress by your favorite designer.

9 *Dare to be different:* When everyone else is wearing a cute little summery dress and flip-flops to the pool party, show up in short-shorts, stilettos, and a bikini top with a glamour puss hairdo and glamour puss makeup. Don't forget the big black Jackie O. sunglasses.

11 *Dare to be silly:* Childhood games rock. Suggest a game of Truth or Dare, Spin the Bottle, 7 Minutes in Heaven, or 20 Questions at the next house party you attend.

12 *Dare to mix it up:* Mix plaids with stripes. Gwen Stefani does, and she rocks.

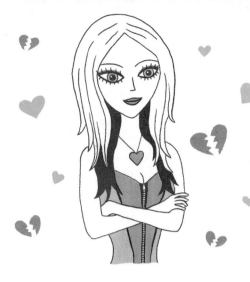

I'm a man—I'm a goddess
I'm a man—Well I'm a virgin
I'm a man—I'm a blue movie
I'm a man—I'm a bitch
I'm a man—I'm a geisha
I'm a man—I'm a little girl
And we make love together."
~BERLIN, "SEX (I'M A . . .)"

DATING, DOING IT & DUMPING

𝕭𝖞 𝕿𝖊𝖗𝖗𝖎 𝕹𝖚𝖓𝖓 𝖔𝖋 𝕭𝖊𝖗𝖑𝖎𝖓

DATING: GETTING THE GUY

"My seduction moves are sort of subtle, but they seem to work. I look at a guy longer than a few seconds—catch his eye—and continuously look back again. If the guy's into me at all, he'll accept this invitation to come over.

Then I use a technique my mom gave me that never fails: "If you want to be interesting, be interested." Ask him questions and listen to the answers. People love talking about themselves, and they'll think you're the greatest person in the world without knowing why (it's more fun for me too; I already know plenty about myself).

But subtlety like this doesn't work very well on rock star guys. Most of the musicians I've dated were too passive for me. I don't know if it's because their feminine side is more developed (making music being a more emotional job than, say, welding). But almost

CHERRY BOMB

every musician I've met told me they got into music for the chicks, so it's like they learned an instrument to court women instead of learning how to court women directly. And hey, it works!

Most of the rock guys I've known are the sit-back-and-wait-for-the-girl-to-come-over type. They play. The girls swoon and throw their room keys on the stage. So to stand out from the crowd, you usually have to get more in their faces to express your interest than you would with the average guy. But avoid putting rock stars on a pedestal. Most sane people want to date equals. Saying you like their music is different than saying, "OH MY GOD! I CAN'T BE-LIEVE I'M TALKING TO YOU!! I'VE BEEN A FAN FOR [fill in number of] YEARS!!! CAN I GET A PICTURE?" Flattering, but not a turn-on.

DOING IT

ROLE-PLAYING

I wrote a whole song about the power of role-playing. "Sex (I'm a . . .)" came about because my boyfriend at the time and I fell into a bit of a rut sexually, so I tried to introduce some role-playing.

After a couple of nights of this, he said, "Terri, I'm not a pirate. I'm not a burglar. I'm just a guy. I just like guy things." Great. If you notice in the song, all he says in the chorus is "I'm a man, I'm a man, I'm a man." BOOOORRRRIINNNNNGG! I'm all kinds of things, a bitch, geisha, blue movie, goddess, virgin. . . . Fuck you! I'm interesting. He laughed at the song, and we did eventually try some more fun scenes in bed.

All guys have their kinks, and role-playing can help bring them out. I've always been fascinated by the fact that you never can tell from looking at a guy what he's really into, deep down. And since men love it when we come, you should do whatever you need to do to come; if that includes role-playing, great. Come as much as possible. Be selfish about it. Include him in any way—a little or completely. He'll be thrilled.

GOOD MORNING!

Men love being woken up with a blow job. It's a slam-dunk every time. I also haven't met a man who doesn't love a girl dancing for him—naked or in any flimsy thing. You don't even have to be a good dancer. Just move any way you want to the music of your choice, and he'll be ecstatic. Especially if he is lying between your legs looking straight up at you dancing over him.

GIRLIE ACTION

Make love to your own sex at least once. Though I discovered that I'm not really even bisexual, it totally changed my life for the better. I discovered how amazing I felt to a guy (she felt amazing!), how awesome my lips must feel (kissing her was completely different than a guy—fantastic!), and how much fun it must be to watch me come (she was incredible!). In short, being a girl rocks, and how else will you ever know this experientially? I didn't expect this extra perk when I did it, but not only was it amazing, it gave me a new sense of self-esteem.

THE MILE-HIGH CLUB

Though I'm not much of an exhibitionist sexually (go figure!), one of the best times I ever had was having sex on a plane. My husband and I threw a blanket over ourselves and started petting heavily. This went on for a while. By the time we locked the bathroom door and he got his dick into me, I came in about three seconds.

KINKY ACTION

Some kind of bondage is worth trying once. Or S&M play where he tells you what to do or vice versa. It's a fun power exchange, and it can be really sexy.

FUN FACT: *Terri Nunn drank apricot brandy in the studio while recording "Sex (I'm a . . .)"* *to help her get in a sexy mood to sing!*

There's nothing wrong with mourning the good times. I'm a solid believer in a good cry. It cleanses the wounds inside and heals the soul. There's strength on the other side of it that makes me a better person.

But it's important for me to remember that what I'm missing when I'm pining away for someone are the good times. Usually a breakup happens after the relationship's been shitty for a while. I have to remind myself that if I got it back, we would be where we left off—shitty. It might never go back to the good times either. You can't go backward, only forward. Then I need to remember that I don't deserve shitty.

If there's more to communicate post-breakup, I try to do it in as loving and honest a way as I can. If he doesn't respond at all or responds in a negative way, all the more reason to get out and stay out. If there's willingness on both sides to work on it, and a reasonable belief that it might turn around, great.

If it's irreparable, lean on girlfriends. Lovers will come and go, but girlfriends are forever. True ones, anyway. Let it all out with them, even the irrational stuff. Let your girlfriends know if you just want them to listen and support you or give you loving feedback. I could not make it in this world without my girlfriends.

DATING QUIZ:

So, You Want to Date a Rock Star?

Sure, rocker boys are cute and sexy, mysterious and danger- ous, wild and unfailingly cool. That's why we love them.

But why should one love *you*? You might think you want to rock his world by being his girlfriend, his muse, or his best lover ever (good luck on that!). But do you have what it takes to get past a first meet- ing? A certain look, a certain attitude, and a certain *je ne sais quoi* can go a long way, but it's not always that easy to actually live in their world. Not every girl can date a creative creature like this. They have special needs, and it takes a very special person to truly understand those needs.

This quiz will give you the reality check you might need to see if you should steer clear of rocker boys, tidy up your act to go from a one-night stand to a blissful rock wife or girlfriend, or verify that you've been doing it right all along.

Get your pens out, ladies.

① You win backstage passes to your favorite band's show. The drummer is single and cute and you want to say hi. Okay, let's be real: You want to jump his skinny rock star bones. How do you approach him?

a. You politely linger near him—but not too close—and wait for him to notice you and make the first move.

b. Musicians love bold women, right? Yoko Ono and Courtney Love sure knew how to dominate a room. You take the lead, march right up to him, give him your number, say, "I think you're cute," and walk away.

c. You find the right time to get closer to him and have a simple conversation. If he's going to get a beer, you go get a beer too, then catch his eye and casually introduce yourself. If it's meant to be, he'll keep the conversation going.

② When a rocker boy asks you, "What music do you like?" you answer . . .

a. I love all music. I listen to everything. Really. Pop, rock, hip-hop, etc. I just love music.

b. Honestly, YOUR band is my favorite band. Look. I have a tattoo of your band's name on my butt cheek.

c. Without skipping a beat, you rattle off the top five songs on your iPod.

③ Which song best describes you?

a. Gnarls Barkley's "Crazy"

b. Beyoncé's "Crazy in Love"

c. Patsy Cline's "Crazy"

④ Which rock star girlfriend best describes you?

a. Penny Lane, Kate Hudson's character in *Almost Famous*

b. Emily Poule, Jennifer Aniston's character in *Rock Star*

c. Jeanine Pettibone, June Chadwick's character in *This Is Spinal Tap*

5 Your boyfriend agreed to escort you to your third cousin's wedding, which will be his debut with your family. But his band gets a last-minute gig—that is TWO weeks away—and they want to rehearse on the wedding night. What do you do?

a. You remind him what a talented, fabulous musician he is and that missing one band practice when there are many more he can attend in the next weeks won't kill him.

b. It's just your third cousin. Go to the wedding alone and deal with it.

c. You have to put your foot down. Tell him he needs to stick to his commitments. He promised you first.

6 Your boyfriend invites you out to a band dinner after the show. They all want to go for sushi. You hate sushi. In fact, you're allergic. You . . .

a. Whine "But I hate sushi" and whimper a bit in that sex-kitten way of yours until the band members change their minds.

b. Pair off. Make your boyfriend take you somewhere else. You need your alone time together anyway.

c. Keep quiet about your aversion to raw fish, go along with the guys, and order a salad.

7 It's concert day. Which best describes how you experience his show?

a. You bring your gaggle of girlfriends and party down. You and your friends are the band's number one fans. You sing along and cheer loudly in the crowd.

b. You buddy up to the singer's wife/girlfriend and do whatever she says.

c. You show restrained support by watching from the front of the house, clapping when a song ends.

8 The girlfriend or wife of another bandmate is being bitchy to you. What do you do?

   a. Don't let her see you sweat. Bite your tongue. Suck it up. Find that inner strength you know you have. You are there for your man, not to make friends.

   b. Have a heart-to-heart with your boyfriend about having a heart-to-heart with the bandmate of the bitchy broad. He should intervene and help smooth things over.

   c. You can't help it. She's so mean, you just start crying.

9 Girls love your man as much as you do. You knew this going in, but you still can't stand to see the groupies flirting with your guy. How do you handle it?

   a. Let the wannabe flirt and let your man enjoy it a little bit. But be sure to cozy up to him, lock your finger into his belt hoop, and stare her down. She can flirt, but she needs to know that he is taken.

   b. This would never happen because you already have a prearranged agreement with your man about not getting into these situations.

   c. Be cool to her. Tell her you like her shoes. Kill her with compliments. Once she knows you're not threatened, she knows she doesn't have a shot and your man will be impressed by your coolness.

10 You check out your boyfriend's band's MySpace page and read a comment from DrummerLover69 that says, "Thanks for last night! Let's do it again." Uh, your boyfriend said he was in band practice last night. What do you do?

   a. Nothing. You didn't read it because you make it a point NOT to read anything online about your boyfriend or his band. Nothing good can come of it.

CARRIE BORZILLO-VRENNA

No

52

b. Naturally, you get all Samuel L. Jackson on her and post a message saying, "Get Your Mother F-ing Hands Off My Mother F-ing Man!" Then you grill your man until he fesses up.

c. You ask him if he's cheating on you. Who is this girl? Does he know her? You deserve to know!

$CORING

1	**a.** 2 points **b.** 1 point **c.** 3 points
2	**a.** 2 **b.** 1 **c.** 3
3	**a.** 3 **b.** 1 **c.** 2
4	**a.** 3 **b.** 2 **c.** 1
5	**a.** 2 **b.** 3 **c.** 1
6	**a.** 1 **b.** 2 **c.** 3
7	**a.** 2 **b.** 1 **c.** 3
8	**a.** 3 **b.** 1 **c.** 2

CHERRY BOMB

⑨	**a.** 1 **b.** 2 **c.** 3
⑩	**a.** 3 **b.** 1 **c.** 2

ℜESULTS

If your score is 1–10, then you are one CRAZY BITCH. Groupie? Perhaps. Rock star girlfriend? Not quite yet. Why? You party too much. You're bossy. You're a bit crazy and way too unpredictable. That might have worked for Yoko Ono and John Lennon, but look what happened there. You can't be the center of attention or demanding when you're in his world.

If your score is 11–20, then you are one SWEET CHILD O'MINE, like a golden retriever puppy that rolls over and bellies up for a tummy rub from a stranger. But your personality is more appropriate for the Timid Dog section in the dog park of rock and roll. You're just too sweet for rock and roll, baby!

If your score is 21–30, then you are one kick-ass KILLER QUEEN. Welcome to the club, you divine rocker chick you! You ARE rock star girlfriend material. You got it right. You know when to hold them, know when to fold them, know when to walk away, and know when to run.

BONUS POINTS: Who performed the songs "Crazy Bitch," "Sweet Child O' Mine," and "Killer Queen"?

ANSWERS: Buckcherry, Guns N' Roses, and Queen

DOLCE & GABBANA

What Makes Dolce & Gabbana Rock?

From rock and pop to R&B and hip-hop, Dolce & Gabbana's appeal crosses musical genres with their sexy and strong femme fatale looks. It's clothing for women who know how to crack a whip but also know how to be in touch with their softer, feminine sides—women like Madonna and Angelina Jolie.

The Italian duo—Domenico Dolce (born September 13, 1958, in Palermo, Sicily, Italy) and Stefano Gabbana (born November 14, 1962, in Venice, Italy)—are the hotshots responsible for the provocative costumes of Madonna's 1993 "The Girlie Show" tour, which ranged from black shorts and a sequined bra paired with dominatrix boots to a Victorian-inspired outfit to a simple white tank top and cutoff jean shorts. Dolce & Gabbana also outfitted Whitney Houston for her 1999 "My Love Is Your Love" tour, which featured an array of bustier bras with animal prints and sequins, and they've designed tour outfits for Beyoncé, Missy Elliott, and Mary J. Blige, among others.

Iconic tour costumes aside, Dolce & Gabbana's most famous looks and trends are their corset dresses (which show off their favorite

CHERRY BOMB

form: the hourglass figure), underwear as outerwear, animal prints (leopard, python, and tiger), pinstriped suits for men, and mixing masculine and feminine influences, such as pairing a more manly gray herringbone tweed with girlie black lace trim for a smoking hot suit. It's all about the supreme sexiness of rock and roll for this dynamic fashion duo.

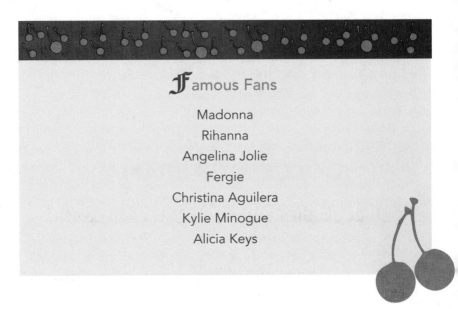

Famous Fans

Madonna
Rihanna
Angelina Jolie
Fergie
Christina Aguilera
Kylie Minogue
Alicia Keys

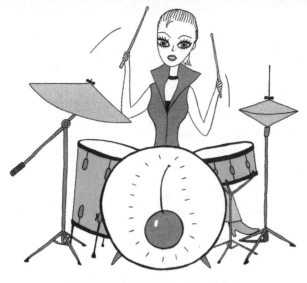

DRUM LESSON

By Samantha Maloney of Peaches

Say you are on your first or second date with a guy. He brings you back to his house for another drink and proceeds to show you around the place. Oh dear! What's that you spot over there in the corner? Is that a drum set? Now, there are many thoughts that can enter your mind. Are his parents sleeping upstairs? Does he have a younger sibling living with him? Is he fulfilling a childhood fantasy? Is he in a local bar band? Does he merely dabble in percussion? Is he a soon-to-be rock star? All of a sudden, stupid drummer jokes come to mind. (What do you call a drummer who breaks up with his girlfriend? *Homeless*.)

Whatever the case, there is no denying that there is going to be a person sitting behind the kit within the next thirty seconds. Drums are funny that way. They are magnets for people with musical talent and for those without. People see them and have an uncontrollable urge that draws them straight to the skins. Whether it is a primal urge to beat the shit out of something and walk away guilt-free or a fascination with the idea of playing an instrument that seems oh so familiar, fun and easy, one never gives up the chance to sit behind the set. And you should be no exception.

CHERRY BOMB

All this being said, herein lies the absolute. Are you going to pass the test and be able to play a beat? Sociocultural studies on this topic have shown that nine out of ten times a woman will most annoyingly fail the test. Two out of ten women can't even hold a drumstick properly. Okay, so this was my own little study conducted by me, but you get the point. It's time to see if you can pass the drum test, and this means so much more than playing a beat.

When a guy sees that a girl can pick up drumsticks with confidence and play a beat, there are many facets to this rare occurrence. First, it is very sexually suggestive. You know how to hold a stick. You know how to use all four limbs at the same time. You like to take control. Second, it shows that you are down with the idea of playing an instrument deemed taboo for a girl by yesteryear's standards. And that in itself rocks. The drum is a physical instrument, and most men, with their small brains, can't fathom a chick throwing down a beat. And last, but definitely not least, it shows the boys that you can hang.

I must admit: I never picked up a drumstick to impress a boy. I am obsessed with music and how it makes me feel. Most drummers are great dancers, which makes sense, because we FEEL what most people just HEAR—the beat. And it makes us move. Like the moon controls the tides, the drummer controls the way the music feels. Drummers control how you move . . . be it at a rock concert, a dance club, listening to a hip-hop song on a radio station, or even sulking in your bedroom listening to PJ Harvey. And I'm going to make sure you know how to feel and control the beat.

So here's a quick little drum lesson for you ladies. Whether you are trying to impress that hot guy with the drum set while on a hot date or getting ready to start your own band (see Warning on page 61), the result will be the same—an amazing sense of accomplishment and a pretty good ego boost to boot.

SETTING UP SHOP

1 Find a drum set. Maybe your cousin Leonard has one in his basement or your best friend's boyfriend is a drummer. Maybe you could go to your local music school and ask to rent a drum room for an hour. The drum set you find is most likely going to be set up as a right-handed drummer's drum set. If you are a lefty, you can still learn how to play drums this way—the right way—pun intended.

2 Get a few pairs of drumsticks. You can find these at your local music store. If the misogynist store clerk asks you if you are buying sticks for your boyfriend, kindly tell him, "No, I am buying them for YOUR boyfriend." Try out different sticks and see what feels most comfortable. I use Zildjian Super 5b wood-tip. 5b is an industry-standard-size stick.

Sometimes sticks have plastic tips at the end. I don't recommend these, as they can fall off and remind me of that line in the movie *A Christmas Story*—"You'll shoot your eye out!"

HERE'S HOW TO PROPERLY HOLD YOUR STICKS: Make sure the bottom of the stick is lying somewhere around the far corner of your hand a few inches underneath your pinky, opposite the base of your thumb. Grip the stick with the first third of your forefinger and the fingerprint on your thumb. Gently wrap your three remaining fingers around the stick loosely.

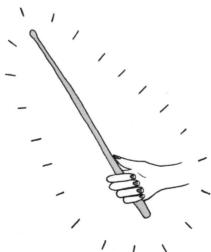

3 I suggest buying a rudiment pad so you can practice paradiddles, flams, and ratamacues. These are all "rudiments" in a drummer's hand vocabulary. A rudiment is a stick pattern played at a certain metronomic speed of your choice to practice and later apply to the drum set. For example, a paradiddle is the stick pattern RLRR LRLL (Right Left Right Right / Left Right Left Left).

4 Get the drum stool set up to your height. Not any little chair will do. You need a proper drum stool that moves with you and fits your crotch and butt nicely.

𝔄 BASIC BEAT

1 We're going to start with the hi-hat. The hi-hat is on the stand to your left, which has two cymbals facing each other. Put your left foot on the hi-hat pedal. When you press down hard with your left foot on the hi-hat pedal, the hats close. When you release your foot, the hats stay open. Now stomp down on the hi-hat pedal eight times in a row at the same speed. Keep doing that without stopping for twenty seconds. You are now "keeping time."

2 Put your right foot on the bass drum pedal. This is the pedal that connects to the bass drum (also known as the kick drum). The bass drum is the biggest drum and is arguably the most important part of the set.

3 Now that you have your feet on the proper pedals, I want you to stop and see if your knees are bent so that your legs are at a 45-degree angle. If they are bent any more or less than that, you must stop and adjust your drum stool appropriately.

4 The next drum you will be hitting—this time with a drumstick—is the snare drum. The snare drum should be sitting between both of your legs. It is the drum with metal strands (aka, snares) underneath that when tightened give the drum a crisp, cracking, poplike sound to it.

Warning: *Drums are LOUD. Cymbals are even LOUDER. Ear piercing, in fact. Proceed with caution. If you start a band, wear earplugs when you play. I cannot play without them.*

5 Go ahead, play. See how easy it is? Ha! Just kidding. Some of us are born with rhythm, and others have to practice hard to find the rhythm inside them. Don't be discouraged. Practice makes [Neil] Peart-fect. (That's a dumb drum joke I just made up. Neil Peart is a master drummer from the highly acclaimed prog-rock band Rush, who to this day is rocking beats that Stephen Hawking has yet to discover. If you want to play drums or even date a drummer, you need to know who Neil Peart is.)

GETTING YOUR GROOVE ON

1 Okay, now let's get you playing that beat. I want you to close your hi-hat with your left foot. Hold it down tight with your foot so you get a nice crisp "chik" when you strike the hi-hat with your right stick with a quick wrist motion (like a nun would strike a child with a ruler or how a dominatrix cracks the whip on her submissive). Now try this: Count in time steadily (meaning don't rush or slow down) from 1 to 8. When you get to 8, start counting again from the top, 1-2-3-4-5-6-7-8, like it is your mantra. To keep time properly, start by taking it nice and slow. Try the 1-Mississippi, 2-Mississippi method like you did as a child when you'd play hide-and-seek.

2 Start hitting the tightly closed hi-hat on every 1 to 8 count (whether you are counting in your head or out loud) with your right stick in your right hand. With your left hand, get ready to hit the snare drum on the 3 and 7 of your count. Don't forget to keep playing the hi-hat with your right hand nonstop and in time.

CHERRY BOMB

3 Next, on every 3 and 7, hit the snare drum with your left stick with a confident whipping of the wrist motion. After you hit the snare on the 3, bring the stick up a bit so you will be ready to hit the snare again for the 7 count. Do this for a minute until you have it down. If you mess up, just stop, regroup, breathe, and think. You can do this. Now, try it again.

4 Once you are rocking this, it is a sure thing that you will get ahead of yourself and strike any drum or cymbal in sight in an attempt to think you can now master a $\frac{5}{4}$ drum fill. This is sure to bring you back to the reality that you need to fully accomplish a basic beat before you set your sights on creating your own version of Alex Van Halen's "Hot for Teacher" drum solo.

5 So, back to the basics. You are playing the hi-hat 1-2-3-4-5-6-7-8 and you are also playing the snare drum on the 3 and the 7. Now we are going to bring in the big Kahuna—the bass drum. You are going to press down with a fervent force on that kick drum pedal on the 1 and 5 of your 8 count. Don't rush. Don't hurt yourself. Just relax and play with confidence. You are gonna get it in no time.

6 After a minute of doing this nonstop, you will get that OMG feeling. You are doing it!! You are playing a beat! You are playing drums! Now what? Start singing AC/DC's" "Back in Black," the Talking Heads' "Take Me to the River," Hall & Oates'"Private Eyes," Men at Work's "Who Can It Be Now?" Survivor's "Eye of the Tiger," or a slew of other songs, because they all carry this same basic beat. This is the basic beat that every drummer needs to get their rock and roll fantasy started!

Good job!

So, you want to start a band?

First, check out the Four Tips to Live (and Rock) By from Jessicka, who has fronted such indie bands as Jack Off Jill, scarling., and the Ingénues.

TIP 1: **Bands are like marriages. You need to pick bandmates that you really want to be with for richer or for poorer (usually poorer), better or for worse, in (dope) sickness and in (mental) health, and till death (or loss of record contract) do you part. To minimize friction within the group, only take on members you absolutely need and connect with. Take on too many people, and it's like telling more than one person you'll go to the prom with them. The end results aren't going to be pretty, and you could get punched in the face. This step will ultimately decide your level of happiness, creativity, chances of success, and ability to leave behind a legacy. Choose wisely.**

TIP 2: **What's in a name? Oh, just about everything. Picking a band name is not easy, and it *is* a very big deal. Your name needs to represent you as a band or, at the very least, look awesome on a T-shirt. Your band name is the brand, and your music is the product. Make them both recognizable and memorable, and you are off to a great start.**

TIP 3: **Spread your name around and don't be shy about it. Talk it up to everyone, create a simple website (or take advantage of MySpace's free hosting services for bands), and create eye-catching fashion-forward merchandise that people will want to wear and thus help in spreading the word. Get stickers made and stick them where the sun don't shine—club bathrooms, back of cars, other bands' guitar cases, etc. In this day and age, anyone can utilize both guerilla and viral marketing as powerful weapons in the fight to get both their name and music out to the general public.**

TIP 4: Play your asses off. If you can't book a proper gig, play your friend's birthday party for free, play college parties, hell, play the Laundromat (some serve beer). Just play and get experience. Videotape your gigs so you can see what works and what doesn't; if the performance is good enough, send the tape to clubs to get more gigs. If you truly bomb or something embarrassing happens (like your singer pees herself onstage like Fergie did or the drummer threw up over nerves), you can capitalize on your embarrassment by getting the video up on YouTube and creating buzz for yourself. (Remember—any press is good press.)

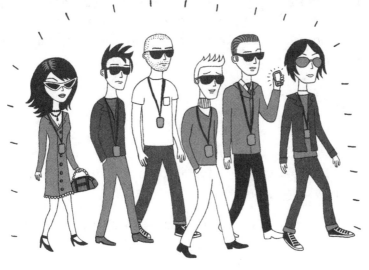

ENTOURAGES

Here's the scenario: You just started dating a celebrity or you've palled up with a famous friend. It's your first big night out with the celeb—an awards show, a concert, or just a night out at the clubs. Things happen fast, and no one can really prepare you for the mayhem that might ensue while you are cruising through a club or the streets of la la land rolling twenty-deep. How do you stay cool and seem like you've been doing this for-e-ver?! Don't fret, just follow this advice:

1 Don't smile. That's not cool. But don't snarl either. That's not nice.

2 Wear oversized sunglasses even if you're indoors or it's nighttime.

3 Don't wave to the cameras or react to cries of "I love you!" or "You suck!"

4 Follow whomever you are with. Your place is behind the hotshots, not next to them or in front of them.

5 Hold your head up, but don't make eye contact with the on-lookers.

CHERRY BOMB

6 Be securely fastened before you start walking. Make sure your shoes are tied and your purse is zipped up, because there is nothing more embarrassing than holding up a posse because you're on the ground collecting the contents of your spilled purse.

7 Don't talk on your cell phone.

8 Don't snap pictures of the chaos around you.

9 If you are taking up the rear of the entourage, don't be TOO far behind, because you might not make it through that elevator or limo you're following your buddy into.

10 Do whatever the leader of the pack asks you to do within reason.

ENTRANCES

Making a grand entrance (or at least a confident entrance) is all about style, grace, panache, and a cool, calm, and collected disposition with a little air of owning the place mixed in. Here are a few pointers on entering that bar, restaurant, or party alone that don't involve talking on your cell phone or texting away like mad until your friend shows up.

■ Before you leave your house, have coffee, tea, or an energy drink to keep yourself UP instead of low.

■ Right before walking through that door, adjust yourself. Make sure your jacket is tied, your purse is zipped, and your lip gloss is glistening.

■ Walk with a purpose with your head held high and your shoulders back.

■ Casually wink at the first guy you see to get your sassy mojo going. If he's not cute and he takes that wink as an invitation to hit on you, you can just say you had an eyelash in your eye. But at least it'll give you someone to talk to right away while you wait for your friend. If he is cute, then it's really a win-win situation.

■ March straight up to the bar, order a drink, and chat up the bartender. When the bartender asks, "How are you?" most people reply, "Okay." Or they groan about the weather or something. Surprise him and answer, "I'm fucking fantastic." Make eye contact and smile. That should lead to a conversation, and before you know it your friend will show up.

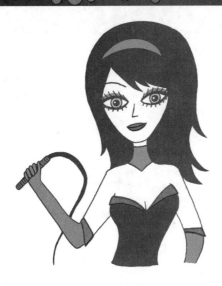

FETISHES

What used to be thought of as someone's dirty little secret has gone oh-so-mainstream in recent years. Maggie Gyllenhaal scored a Golden Globe nomination for her role in *Secretary*, which was about a couple engaging in a BDSM lifestyle. *Family Guy* even got into the bondage business in an episode with Lois and Peter engaging in some "master and slave" play, complete with latex, zippered masks, and ball-gags. And furries were brought to the forefront with the help of episodes of *C.S.I.* and *Entourage*. Fetish is no longer a bad F word, so forget what you thought about fetishes in the past. And they're not necessarily about sex. In most cases, it's about replacing sex with a little bit of fantasy. And, sure, anything can be a fetish. By *Webster*'s definition, a fetish is simply "an object of unreasonably obsessive attention or regard" or "a non-sexual object that arouses or gratifies sexual desire."

This guide will show you the ins and outs of some of the more popular fetishes in practice today.

	BDSM/S&M	SPLOSHING
SAY WHAT?	BDSM stands for bondage, discipline, sadism, and masochism. S&M is either sadism & masochism or slave & master. Call it what you like, it's about one partner being dominant and the other being submissive, and it's about power or humiliation—depending on who's holding the whip.	It's a full-body food fetish.
SIGNATURE ACTS	Tying up, spanking, paddling, whipping, tickling (aka tickle torture), reprimanding, demeaning, overpowering, teasing.	Sploshing is the act of playing around naked and/or having sex in messy places—in mud, in foam, in paint, in oil. But the most popular MO is in gooey foods like cakes, whipped cream, pies, pudding, and pasta. You name it and sploshers will screw in it.
SHOPPING LIST	Riding crops, handcuffs, blindfolds, collars, restraints, floggers, whips, gags, locks, slappers, paddles, mono-gloves, leather, studs, and ticklers.	Plastic sheets to cover the bed, plastic tarps to cover other surfaces, and your favorite food or substance to splosh around in. It's one of the least expensive fetishes.
MEDIA	Movies: *The Notorious Bettie Page, Secretary, The Night Porter, 9½ Weeks*. Books: Madonna's *Sex*, Dita Von Teese's *Burlesque and the Art of the Teese/Fetish and the Art of the Teese*.	British magazine *Splosh!* and the John Waters film *A Dirty Shame*.
TIPS	Come up with a "safe word" to say when you want the activities to stop. "No" doesn't mean *no* in this practice. (Lois and Peter's safe word was "banana.")	Make sure you're not allergic to something before you play around in it. The moment a rash occurs, head to your doctor.

FURRIES	PONY PLAY	FOOT
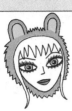	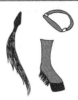	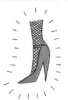
It's a form of "transformation fetishes," where you have sex or just play around while pretending to be an animal.	Another human/animal role-play fetish. Women and men, known as Pony Girls and Pony Boys, dress up as ponies—mostly they're just nude with a harness and plume on, like a show pony. And, no, this is not about Donkey Shows!	The most common fetish is the foot fetish, which involves men being aroused by women's feet and/or seeing feet in extreme shoes.
Having sex while dressed up in your furry costume, acting like the animal you are portraying, pawing and chasing each other like animals.	One participant is the pony; the other is the rider or trainer. They ride each other, walk the "animal," feed them treats, and train them.	Stand naked over your man in a killer pair of shoes or boots, step on him with the boot as a way to assert your dominance, make him lick your shoe or drink champagne out of your shoe, have sex in your shoes only, and pose for Polaroids while lying on your belly holding your heels as if hog-tied.
Head-to-toe stuffed animal costume with a hole or opening in the crotch. The most popular animals for this fetish are the cute and fuzzy ones like foxes, puppies, bunnies, kitties, bears, or chipmunks.	Bit gags, plumes, reins, blinkers, bridles, blinders, saddles, harnesses, butt plugs with tails, pony boots with hooves.	Platform stilettos, pumps, boots at least six inches high. Terrence de Havilland makes killer platforms. You can also ask your local stripper where she got her heels.
Episodes of *C.S.I.*, *Entourage*, *Tori & Dean: Inn Love.* *Yarf!* magazine.	2005 documentary film *Born in a Barn*, Madonna's 2006 "Confessions" tour costumes, Goldfrapp's "Train" music video.	The *Sex and the City* episode "La Douleur Exquise" made Charlotte York the object of attraction of a shoe salesman with a foot fetish. Film director Quentin Tarantino has also reportedly admitted to having a foot fetish.
If you partake in this, you need to create a separate furry persona called a "fursona."	If you have a bad back, don't let someone heavier than you be the rider.	Some shoes are made for walking. Some shoes are made to wear when you're on your back. Confuse the two, and you could suffer a broken ankle!

THE PLEASURE CHEST IN LOS ANGELES, NEW YORK, AND CHICAGO AND ONLINE (WWW.THEPLEASURECHEST.COM) CAN HELP YOU GEAR UP FOR MOST OF THESE FETISHES.

FLIRTING

*A*dmit it, sometimes flirting is better than sex. There is nothing like the magic of the first time you catch a sexy guy's eye and have a playful tête-à-tête. The sexual tension! The excitement of something new! The thrill of the chase!

Flirting is also a great way to get in touch with your inner sexiness, boost your confidence, and help you get through that time in your life between a breakup and when you're actually ready to date again. It can land you a hot date for the upcoming weekend or just help you get your feet wet again in the dating pool.

By the time they hit seventeen, most girls know the basics of flirting. The Flirting 101 moves are simple: Lean in when you talk to him. Listen to what he says and ask questions. Laugh at his jokes—but not every joke. No one is *that* funny. Make good eye contact. Smile. Touch his arm or shoulder once or twice when making a point. And throw in a little teasing or a playful dig to keep him on his toes.

Got that? Okay, here are a few more moves to make on that man before striking up a conversation with him:

THREE FLIRTING MOVES THAT ARE THE (CHERRY) BOMB!

MOVE 1: THE OVER-THE-SHOULDER GLANCE: Move your left shoulder forward and up a bit and stretch your head to the left so your chin is almost resting on that shoulder and you are looking way over your left shoulder. With your best Bette Davis eyes, take a good, long, sexy look at the target of your affection. Bat your eyelashes once and turn away.

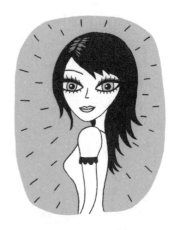

MOVE 2: THE PERFECTLY TIMED YAWN-SLASH-STRETCH: Nothing makes a body look leaner and sexier than stretching it out as far as possible. It's also a good way to stick your bosom out a bit. In this move, you may need to feign exhaustion, but it'll help him get a good look at your best assets. Take your arms over your head, grab one wrist with the other hand, and yawn and stretch as he's looking your way.

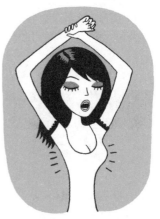

MOVE 3: THE MOUTHING OFF MOVE: Guys love women's mouths. So work those lips and that tongue of yours, girls. Play with the straw in your drink. Lick your lips. Eat cherries from the bar seductively. Hey, you learned how to tie a cherry stem with your tongue on page 9, put your new trick to use! Suck on that celery stick in your Bloody Mary a bit. Put your lipstick on in front of him. (Miss Manners might say it's

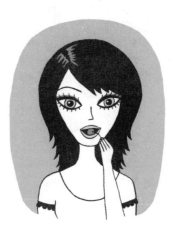

CHERRY BOMB

uncouth to put lipstick on in public, but if you can look hot doing it, go for it!) If you happen to be in a place where an ice cream cone, a Popsicle, or a lollipop are at your service, then you've hit the jackpot of "Mouthing Off" devices. Basically, do anything with your mouth in a seductive way and you're likely to get a rise out of him.

Now that you have the body language going, it's time to strike up that first conversation. Hopefully, if you rocked those moves to their fullest, he's introduced himself to you by now. But if he's a little slow on the uptake, you might need to make the first verbal move. Here's what to do next:

CONVERSATION STARTERS

Guys LOVE it when a girl starts the conversation. Just ask my husband.

True Story: Thank God for Bold Babes!

I'M NOT ASHAMED TO ADMIT IT: I have no game. I've never been one of those guys who would approach pretty strangers. Thank God my wife is the type of woman who isn't afraid to march right up and say hi. That is how our first conversation started. It was more of a business talk, she being a writer and me someone she's written about. But it turned into a personal conversation and ended up with me asking her out. If she didn't come up to me that night, we might not be together today. Guys love it when a woman initiates things—guys always have that fear of rejection but are always expected by society to start first, so any man would love a woman who takes that pressure off of them and starts the conversation first.

~Chris Vrenna

Being the first to initiate a conversation doesn't have to be as scary as it may seem. Think about how often you talk to strangers on a daily basis. You ask for directions or the time regularly, right? There's only one difference between doing that and flirting: If you ask a hot guy who you're interested in "Do you know what time it is?" you need to show him you're not just a time-challenged stranger but you're talking to him because you like him. You do that by rocking some of those flirty moves you just read about— remember to smile, look him seductively in the eye, touch his arm, linger on his gaze a bit, toss the hair away from your face, or chew on that cherry. Now that you have your opening, the best way to start a conversation is to ask a question about the situation you're both in.

SOME SCENARIOS

AT A CONCERT: You can easily strike up a conversation with the guy sitting next to you, in front of you, in back of you, at the concessions stand, anywhere at a concert, because you both already have something in common and something you can talk about right off the bat—the band you're seeing! An easy opener here would be, "Hey, do you know if they played the new single yet? I was in the restroom and I think I missed it." Or "I got here late. What song did they start with?" Use the flirty basics as outlined earlier, and if the chemistry is there, the conversation will continue. After he answers, jump in with a, "Hi, I'm [name]." Then smile and act cute.

AT A BAR: It's a lot easier to introduce yourself to a stranger if you don't have to make that nervous walk across a bar, club, or venue. So after you spot the guy, casually work your way closer to where he's hanging out. Don't make eye contact as you're walking to him, and once you get there, don't immediately jump into his conversation. Instead, just hang and talk with your friends. Get settled before diving in. Once you're nice and relaxed and in position, *then* work in some of that eye contact, smiling, and other body-language moves. THEN lean over and ask him a simple question like "Hey,

CHERRY BOMB

this is my first time here. Do you know if they serve food?" Or, "Is there a smoking patio?" or "Do you know where the restroom is?" Again, after he answers, simply introduce yourself and keep the flirty moves up.

AT A PRIVATE HOUSE PARTY: If you're at a house party and you're friends with the host, you should just have that pal introduce you to the object of your affection. If that's not happening, then take it upon yourself. You can go up to him, touch him gently on the arm to get his attention, and say, "Hey. I have a quick question." Lean in, cup his ear with your hand (hopefully you smell pretty, and if not, then go invest in some perfume!) and say, "Who is that girl over there. I know I know her but I forget her name." After he answers, you can introduce yourself and ask how he knows the host. Or say something playful about how you have an awful memory or beg him not to tell the girl you asked about that you forgot her name. Any of those moves should get the party rolling for you two . . . if he's interested. If he's not, then move on.

AT A DANCE CLUB: If you're feeling bold, march up to the cute guy, introduce yourself, and ask him if he wants to dance. If that's too much, then you can ask him if he knows the name of the song that's playing right now or who the DJ is. Throw in a few flirty moves and chat him up. If he takes you up on your invitation to hit the dance floor, dance like you're having fun, slightly seductively, and don't forget to make eye contact and rub up against him once in a while.

$\mathcal{F}$LIRTING THE FRENCH WAY

Nothing is sexier than the sound of the French language. It is a language of love, after all. And men dig French girls. Master these lines from a few cool songs and save them for the END of your night of flirting with him.

1 "Oo, appelle-moi mon cherie, appelle-moi," from Blondie's "Call Me." Translation? "Call me, my darling."

2 "Voulez-vous coucher avec moi (ce soir)?" from Patti LaBelle's "Lady Marmalade" (made all the more sexier in 2001 by Christina Aguilera, Lil' Kim, Mya, and Pink). Translation? "Do you want to sleep with me (tonight)?"

3 [Insert your man's name here] and then say, "Ma belle. Sont des mots qui vont très bien ensemble," from the Beatles'"Michelle." Translation? "Michelle, my beautiful. These are the words that go together well."

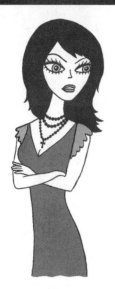
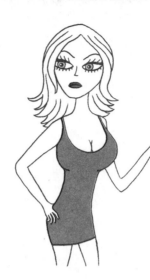

"When you were down they were never there,
When you're all alone you really get to learn,
If you get back up they gonna come around,
All the sycophants they love to make romance,
To the ugly sound of 'em tellin' you what you wanna hear an' you pretend."

~JOAN JETT & THE BLACKHEARTS, "FAKE FRIENDS"

FRIENEMIES

Popularized in the Lindsay Lohan movie *Mean Girls* in 2004, frienemy is a mash-up of *friend* and *enemy*. Whether we like it or not, frienemies enter our lives like Tasmanian devils and can cause quite a stir. The goal is to identify them and kick them to the curb as fast as you can say *"Oh no you didn't!"* It's not so easy to identify a fake friend, or friendly enemy, when her dis is coupled with a compliment or when that dig comes with a smile. Frienemies seduce you into a false sense of friendship and then hit you when you're least expecting it just to feel better about themselves or take advantage of what you have to offer.

The following examples should help you figure out if you've made a friend or a frienemy:

She's your friend if she holds your hair back while you throw up after a night of partying like a rock star. She's your frienemy if she does so while secretly snapping a picture from her camera phone.

She's your friend if you coordinate outfits before a big night out. She's your frienemy if she tells you she's wearing jeans and boots and shows up in a cute little minidress and stilettos.

CARRIE BORZILLO-VRENNA

She's your friend if she points out that your boobs look bigger. She's your frienemy if she tells you, "You look like you've gained weight. But it looks great in your boobs!"

She's your friend if she marvels at the new rock on your finger, congratulates you on the big news, and wants every little detail of the proposal. She's your frienemy if she looks at the ring on your finger and says, "Oh. Your ring is so cute!"

She's your friend if she calls you to share her good news *and* bad news. She's your frienemy if she only calls to brag.

She's your friend if she acts as your wing-woman when you're out trolling for men. She's your frienemy if she slips the guy you're interested in her number instead.

She's your friend if she tells you "You look great!" even when you don't. She's your frienemy if she says, "You look great. You must have lost weight, huh?"

She's your friend if she tells you she saw your boyfriend kissing another girl (and it's the truth). She's your frienemy if she tells you upsetting stuff about your boyfriend's love life that happened years before you ever met him.

She's your friend if she totally understands that you had to cancel plans because you got into a terrible fight with your boyfriend . . . even if those plans were for New Year's Eve. She's your frienemy if all she thinks about is how her night was ruined and then proceeds to air your dirty laundry while she's out.

She's your friend if she tells you how awesome your wedding dress, wedding plans, and wedding hair is. She's your frienemy if she copies everything you did for her own wedding and played it off as if they'd been her original ideas.

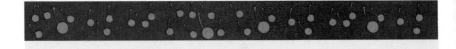

Famous Frienemies

Hilary Duff & Lindsay Lohan
Tyra Banks & Naomi Campbell
Ginger & MaryAnn (*Gilligan's Island*)

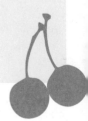

FUNK FIXERS

We've all been there. For whatever reason, we sometimes just fall into a funk that ruins our whole day, weekend, or, heaven forbid, a whole week. Nothing feels better than just curling up on your couch with your furry companion, watching rainy-day movies, eating comfort food (carbs!), and hating everything and everyone.

Indulge in your dark side for a day. But on the next day, it's time to take action. Sitting around moping and watching TV will only sink you further into your funk. Instead, force yourself to do at least one thing on this list to help tweak yourself back into the chipper person you were the week before.

1 Play your favorite music extra loud and sing until your heart's content! Here are some songs that should take you from funk to fun in no time:

"Get the Funk Out," Extreme

"We Got the Funk," Positive Force version

"Give Up the Funk (Tear the Roof Off the Sucker)," Parliament

"Girls Just Want to Have Fun," Cyndi Lauper

"All I Wanna Do," Sheryl Crow
"I Wanna Have Some Fun," Samantha Fox
"I'm So Excited," The Pointer Sisters
"Hella Good," No Doubt

2 Surround yourself with flowers, candles, and soothing incense.

3 Be honest. Call your best girlfriends and tell them you're in a funk and need help getting out.

4 If your willpower is stronger than mine and you don't want to eat junk food, then cook yourself a really fun healthy meal. Splurge a bit at the fancy grocery store and buy a $20 lobster or something you normally wouldn't buy for yourself.

5 Jump on your trampoline. I call it tramping. Don't have a trampoline? Put down the book for a minute and go online to buy one.

6 Take your dog for a walk or get out that laser pointer your cat loves and run around the house with the little critter chasing the red beam.

7 Get some coffee, ROCKSTAR energy drink, or green tea with caffeine in you. It's hard to stay low when you have jolts of caffeine running through your system.

8 Shop! Duh! This should be No. 1 on the list, but I'm hesitant to suggest it because we know what a danger zone this can be. To make sure you don't overshop, leave your house with just $20 in your wallet and buy something pretty and small, like lip gloss or a cute pair of panties that make you feel sexy.

9 Watch a really depressing movie to put your little funk in perspective.

10 It's hard to stay in a funk when you are laughing your ass off. Go see a funny movie or buy a stand-up comedian's DVD or CD and get the belly laughs rolling.

JOHN GALLIANO

What Makes John Galliano Rock?

The first time singer Gwen Stefani was invited to a John Galliano for Christian Dior show, she was brought to tears. Who else but the rock star of fashion could do that? Later, Ms. Hollaback Girl famously went on to wear one of Galliano's most notable dresses—her stunning pink and white wedding dress in 2002—but he'd been a favored designer of rock stars long before that.

After a bumpy start in funding his line, the mustached-maverick (born Juan Carlos Antonio Galliano, November 28, 1960, in Gibraltar) was taken under the fashion wing of Anna Wintour, the famed editor-in-chief of American *Vogue*, who helped him secure a backer for his own collection and a venue for his next show, which featured Kate Moss, Christy Turlington, and Naomi Campbell forgoing their usual five-figure salaries to help him out. The event included only seventeen all-black outfits—very rock and roll of him—as that was the only fabric he could afford, but it secured his fate as one of the most exciting designers of his time.

In the mid-1990s, Galliano was appointed chief designer for

Givenchy Ready to Wear and Haute Couture Collections, where he continued to develop his own rocker image and made the brand more eclectic. The bias-cut dress and narrow tailoring became his signature style.

He then became the new designer for Christian Dior and has been rocking both the John Galliano and Christian Dior collections ever since. Some of his most stand-out creations for the red carpet have been seen on Charlize Theron, who wore a hand-painted, steel green, leather silk satin "scissor" gown to the 2006 Academy Awards and a midnight blue empress silk satin gown to the 2005 Golden Globes, both Dior by John Galliano designs.

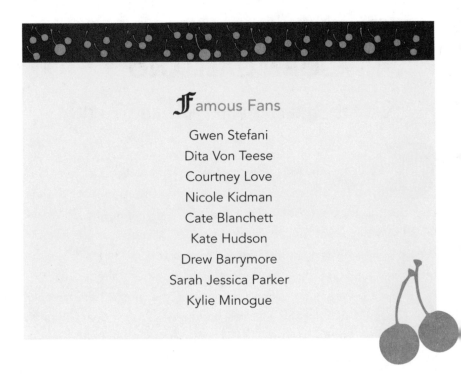

Famous Fans

Gwen Stefani

Dita Von Teese

Courtney Love

Nicole Kidman

Cate Blanchett

Kate Hudson

Drew Barrymore

Sarah Jessica Parker

Kylie Minogue

JEAN-PAUL GAULTIER

What Makes Jean-Paul Gaultier Rock?

Any man who cites such rocking chicks as Joan of Arc, Frida Kahlo, and Nina Simone as influences for his collections gets the rocker chick thumbs-up in my book. (Literally!)

It was Jean-Paul Gaultier's work with Madonna on her "Blond Ambition" tour in 1990 that made the music and fashion worlds take notice. (He was the genius behind her infamous and iconic conical bra. Turning underwear into outerwear with his use of corsets is one of his trademark moves.) Gaultier (born April 24, 1952, in Arcueil, Val-de-Marne, France) later went on to create costumes for Madonna's 2006 "Confessions" tour, including the S&M and equestrian-inspired outfits that people in the fetish world associate with the practice of "pony play."

This bad boy of French fashion (or L'Enfant Terrible, as he's been dubbed) is also known for having fun with traditional male-female roles by using androgynous models. He launched his androgynous collection, A Wardrobe for Two, in 1985, which was the same year he raised eyebrows with his "skirt for men." Another rockin' staple of his

CHERRY BOMB

repertoire at the time was his tattoo-printed shirts and body stockings. A rare misstep was in 1989 when Gaultier dabbled in music, releasing rap song "Ow to Do Zat" ("How to Do That"). It didn't rock. Luckily, he stuck to fashion and has been rocking ever since.

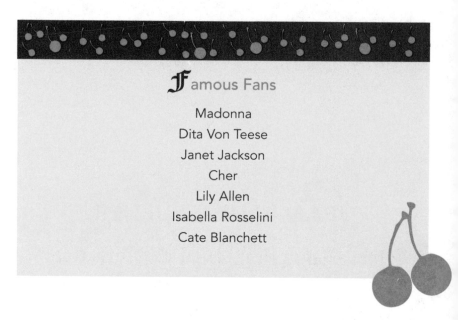

𝔉amous Fans

Madonna
Dita Von Teese
Janet Jackson
Cher
Lily Allen
Isabella Rosselini
Cate Blanchett

GOALS

Sure, there are certain milestones in life we are all expected to reach by a certain age and a number of common goals that most everyone wants to achieve in their lifetime. But with forty being the new thirty and thirty being the new twenty, there's a little wiggle room to have some fun in life too. Long gone are the days when you needed the husband, the house with the white picket fence, the 2.3 kids, the dog, and the shiny new Beamer in the driveway all by age thirty. Try these new goals on for size instead:

OUT: THE YESTERYEAR GIRL GOALS	IN: THE ROCKIN' GIRL GOALS
Join a health club	Join the mile high club
Get a job with a 401(k)	Get a job with season tickets
Save money to buy a house	Save money to buy Christian Louboutin's entire fall collection
Lose weight	Have a healthy mind, body, and soul
Recycle more	Go 100% green
Eat more vegetables	"Veg" out once a week

CHERRY BOMB

OUT: THE YESTERYEAR GIRL GOALS	IN: THE ROCKIN' GIRL GOALS
Find a rich guy	Create your own wealth
Meet a nice guy and settle down	Don't settle for just a nice guy—some "bad boys" are nice too
Be married by age thirty	Be in control of your life by age thirty
Start on the 2.3 kids on your wedding night	Start the baby-making whenever you are damn well ready!

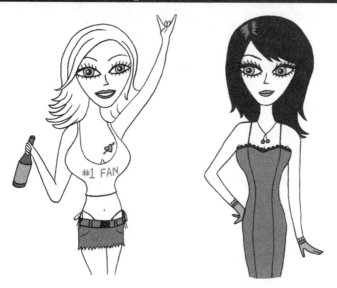

GROUPIE OR GIRLFRIEND?

So, you want to date a boy in a band? Now that you've learned how to sneak backstage, passed the So, You Want to Date a Rock Star? quiz, and are raring to go, what you need to know is that musicians and celebrities have their own personal checklists that help them size you up as either a groupie or a potential girlfriend. And they're assessing you from the moment they meet you until the moment they kick you out of their dressing room, tour bus, or bed.

TELLTALE SIGNS THAT YOU'RE A GROUPIE

1 You wear his band's T-shirt to his show.

2 You offer to service him before even saying hello.

3 You have posters of him on your bedroom ceiling.

4 You have a tattoo of him or his band's logo on your body.

5 You watch the show from front and center and actually think he's singing to you.

CHERRY BOMB

6 You recite back to him obscure facts about his life, his career, and his pets.

7 You are a friend on his MySpace page before you ever meet him.

8 You post comments on his band's message board.

9 His current hit song is your ringtone.

10 You say, "I can't believe I'm on a date with you!" (But instead of "you," you say his first and last name.)

TELLTALE SIGNS THAT YOU ARE GIRLFRIEND MATERIAL

1 He approaches you before you approach him.

2 You aren't overly aggressive when you meet him. You play it cool.

3 Your first words are something simple like "Hi, I'm so-and-so. Great show."

4 You act like you don't care that you're talking to a famous musician.

5 You have something else in common other than your mutual love of him.

6 When he asks you what music you like, you name bands other than his.

7 You have your own kick-ass career (artistic or not) that you are passionate about.

8 You don't suggest a hook-up that night.

9 You end the conversation or walk away first.

10 This is your first time backstage.

GUEST LISTS

Guess what? Getting on a guest list isn't as hard as it seems. Sometimes, all you need to do is ask nicely, work your connections, or have a blog. Try these three tips:

1 *Be Bold:* If you work in any area of the entertainment industry (music, television, film, or even porn), just call up and ask to be put on the list. It depends on who picks up the phone at the club, but there's at least someone kind enough in the office that would say yes.

2 *Barter:* Bartering works. If you're a hairstylist, tattoo artist, massage therapist, or have another cool job, you can offer up a free haircut, some tattoo time, or a massage in exchange for a place on the list.

3 *Blog:* It's a blogger's world. If you have your own blog (it doesn't even have to be well established; it just has to be cool) and you cover shows, just call up and say you're covering the show for your blog, and you're on the list.

HANGOVERS

A cool rocker chick is not a sloppy drunk the night of the party or a hungover mess the morning after. If you follow these simple rules while you're out partying like a rock star, you won't end up puking like an amateur.

HOW TO PREVENT A HANGOVER

1 Never drink on an empty stomach. Eat a decent meal before you go out.

2 Chasers. There are tons of antihangover pills out there, but the one that I tried the day of a marathon partying session was called Chasers, and I swear they worked. It's the only way I can explain how I was able to drink twelve beers (over twelve hours and with about five bottles of water in me) at the Coachella Valley Music & Arts festival one year and emerge unscathed. I took two Chasers before I went out and was up bright and early and feeling no pain the next morning.

3 Drink one eight-ounce glass of water for each alcoholic drink you consume. No exceptions. If it means walking around a bar double-fisted (water in one hand, your alcoholic drink in the other), do it. Dehydration is a big reason why you might wake up feeling like crap the next day.

4 Dance your booty off. The more you dance, the more you sweat (or glisten, if you're lucky), and you'll be oozing out the toxins from your pores all night long.

5 Don't go to bed extremely drunk. Your metabolism slows down when you're sleeping, and that makes it harder for your body to process the alcohol in your system. Doing the following before you go to bed will help you sober up a little bit: Have a bedtime snack. Drink a glass of water and/or a glass of Gatorade. Wash your face. Hide your BlackBerry so you don't drunk-text. Have sex with your man. Take a B-12 vitamin. B-12 has been known to help prevent hangovers.

HOW TO PREVENT A DISASTROUS DAY
AT THE OFFICE THE NEXT DAY

If I know I'm going to be partying my butt off and might not be feeling so sharp when I wake up, I prepare for the next day before I go out. I will pick out an outfit to wear and hang it up—with accessories, shoes, and a bag filled with Advil and a bottle of water. I also set my alarm for the next morning before I go out. And I even get my towels, bathrobe, and slippers out and ready for my morning shower.

HOW TO TREAT A HANGOVER

So, you skipped some of those preventative measures I mentioned and you're hungover. Try this:

1 Eat a greasy meal of carbs and protein. Lisa Loeb swears her grilled cheese sandwiches are a great hangover cure. (See page 98 for the recipe.) I love McDonald's. Both can knock a hangover on its ass.

2 Keep hydrating! Drink water, Gatorade, and/or Pedialyte to replenish those fluids.

3 Take a hot shower. It feels good and helps soothe your aching body and pounding head. And the steam helps release toxins.

CHERRY BOMB

4 If the room is spinning and you feel queasy, try PMS pills or Dramamine.

5 Have morning sex. It won't cure your hangover, but it can help make up for any bad drunken behavior from the night before.

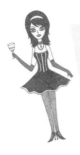

𝕲𝖔𝖙𝖍𝖆 𝕾𝖙𝖊𝖜𝖆𝖗𝖙 𝕿𝖎𝖕: *Drink ginger ale with a few dashes of bitters to help settle an upset tummy. And eat beets regularly. Beets contain antioxidants, and antioxidants have a cleansing effect on the liver. The liver takes a beating when we drink, so eat your beets to help your liver!*

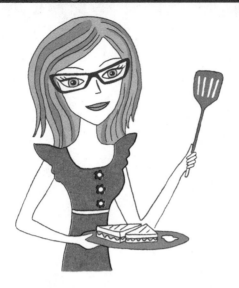

HOSTING 101

By singer-songwriter/foodie Lisa Loeb

"

BE PREPARED: I have pets, so I always ask people if they are allergic to them before they come to my house for a party. If they are, then I warn them that pets will be there and I'll have Claritin-D handy in case they need it. And I make sure I have lint rollers around so people don't leave covered in fur. I also ask if they have any food allergies or if there's anything in particular that they love or don't love or can't eat. I want to always make sure I have things they can eat.

JUST SAY YES: When people ask if they can bring something, I always say yes and have them bring something they like to drink or a dessert. I think of what it's like to be a guest—you want to participate and you want to make sure there is something you really want to eat. If I'm going to a pizza party, I might bring a spinach salad or steamed broccoli or something that balances out what we're going to have. Or if it's going to be a super-healthy party, I might bring the pie. So I encourage my guests to do the same when they come to my house.

CHERRY BOMB

AT YOUR SERVICE: I want my guests to feel comfortable. If there's something they want, I'll get it for them. If there's something they don't like, they don't have to eat it; I'll get them something else. If they spill something, I will clean it up for them. I'm always ready. I have drawers full of cloth napkins and towels. I like being a good hostess. I like feeling useful. I send guests off with doggy bags. It's a very Jewish thing to do. I have a stack of Tupperware, and I push food out the door with people.

WELCOMING NIBBLES: I make sure there is food out when guests arrive. I usually serve things I would eat myself. I like to have a raw vegetable plate so people like me—with a smaller stomach but who also like to eat a lot—have something little to nibble on. I'll do vegetables with guacamole or low-fat sour cream and onion dips. Salsa is always good because it's like not eating food at all, and guests love it. I also have fun stuff like pistachios or dried fruits and berries on hand. I try not to do heavy appetizers so that my guests have room for dinner and dessert.

MIX & MATCH: One of my favorite things to make is my mix-and-match piecrust chips and dips. I like to give people options and give them items in small bites, so I make the piecrusts, and then I make several different fillings or toppings and let my guests choose the combinations they like. As an alternative, you can buy cookies and vanilla wafers and canned fillings and let people put their favorite fillings on their cookies.

CHALLAH-BACK GIRL: I entertain a lot and host a lot of the holidays at my house. I'll have the Jewish holidays, Halloween parties, New Year's Eve, everything. But the parties that my friends love the most are my grilled cheese parties. I have a selection of breads and cheeses—from white bread with American cheese to special thinly sliced challah (pronounced "Holla," a traditional Jewish egg bread) with sharp Cheddar and rosemary on the outside of the bread and a little bit of Parmesan cheese on top so when you cook it on the George Forman grill you get that crisp outer edge. It makes for a great breakfast, lunch, dinner, pool party snack, or game night treat. And it's great for curing a hangover.

QUIRKY COCKTAILING: I like to use up champagne that I get as gifts throughout the year. You don't need to save it for special occasions. I serve it to my guests all the time. I love Veuve Clicquot, and I'll serve it at a weekday lunch with peanut butter and jelly sandwiches. You don't need to serve it with fancy meals only. For summer, a simple, refreshing drink that my friends and I enjoy is vodka, club soda, and a little bit of Rose's lime juice. I always make sure I have plenty of nonalcoholic drinks and water for everyone too. I might serve glasses of water in canning jars, or it's very rock and roll to have water bottles and just use a Sharpie to write your guests' names on them. I do that a lot—it's more fun than using those tags you put on stemware. Besides, at my house, you might be drinking champagne out of a juice glass.

ROCKIN' TABLEWARE: I like to mix and match dishes and put fancy foods on casual plates and casual food on fancy plates. I might serve grilled cheese sandwiches on a fancy plate and then serve fancy food on my McDonald's plastic plates. Those were collector's items for a while in the mid-1990s, and I have a full set of them. I like to use them instead of china. I also collect a lot of dishes from Japan. I have a lot of Hello Kitty dishes and dishes with cute bears or animals with little stars and shapes on them.

CUTTING CALORIES: I serve small portions because I find people are really watching portion sizes these days. So if I put donuts out, I'll put them out with a knife so you can just cut off a bite and not feel like if you want a donut you have to eat the whole thing—same with lasagna and pizza. I cut everything into smaller portions. With pizza, you can make triple cuts to get smaller slices, and then you can try each kind without having to eat full slices of every one. You want to encourage people to eat and try things and not feel like they're stuffing themselves.

NOT SO FAST: My guests might sometimes party like rock stars, but they'll never leave my house in that state of mind. I'll have extra cash on hand in case someone needs to take a cab, or I'll make sure a friend takes him or her home. But most of the people at my parties are my good friends, so they're always welcome to stay over. I'll let

CHERRY BOMB

them sleep it off and sleep in. And I'll be ready for them in the morning with fresh towels, spare deodorant, an extra toothbrush, and, of course, breakfast and coffee.

Lisa Loeb's Crisp-Top Grilled Cheese Sandwiches

1–2 oz. sharp Cheddar or mozzarella cheese

2 slices of fresh challah, thinly sliced (Ask the bakery to slice the bread for you. Thinner slices equals fewer calories and crispier sandwiches.)

1 tsp. olive oil

$\frac{1}{2}$ tsp. fresh rosemary leaves, stems removed

$1\frac{1}{2}$ tbs. fresh grated Parmesan cheese

Cut the Cheddar or mozzarella into $\frac{1}{4}$-inch-thick slices.

Lightly brush one side of each piece of bread with the olive oil or pour the oil onto a clean plate and mop it up with one side of each piece of bread.

Place the oiled side of the bread onto a George Forman grill (a panini sandwich maker will also work).

Add the slices of cheese on top of the bread.

Cover the sandwich with another piece of bread, making sure the oiled side is up and exposed to the grill.

Combine the rosemary and Parmesan and sprinkle the mixture over the top of the sandwich.

Close the grill and cook until the cheese is melted and the bread is crispy and golden.

To complete the meal, plate the sandwich with a side of Dijon mustard for dipping and serve with a fresh spinach salad.

Lisa Loeb's recipe was created with the help of Chef Dawn Roznowski from Full Plate.

> *Don't cha wish your girlfriend was a freak like me?"*
> ~THE PUSSYCAT DOLLS, "DON'T CHA"

HOTTER GIRLFRIEND IN 30 DAYS:
A Calendar

Don't let this song happen to you. Avoid having some freaky, sexy, raw, fun chick get all up in your man's grill: Be that freaky, sexy, raw, fun chick yourself.

Sometimes being a hot girlfriend means putting aside your feminist ways just for a night and letting his manly needs come first. You might need to bend over backward to get what you want in the end. Try out the following selfless acts of love and see what happens. Chances are, your cool and oh-so-eager-to-please ways will keep him in line and more willing to serve you in a similar way in the near future. Tit for tat, so to speak.

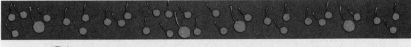

The Hottest Rock Star Girlfriends & Wives

Priscilla Presley (Elvis Presley)
Bianca Jagger (Mick Jagger)
Anita Pallenberg (Keith Richards)
Patricia Keneally (Jim Morrison)
Bebe Buell (Steven Tyler, Todd Rundgren)

CHERRY BOMB

SUNDAY	MONDAY	TUESDAY	WEDNESDAY	THURSDAY	FRIDAY	SATURDAY
1 Don't interrupt him while he's watching the game. In fact, bring him a beer in a low-cut shirt, bend over to give it to him, and treat him to a sweet peck on the lips.	2 Let him have "a case of the Mondays" without asking "What's wrong??! Is it me???" every two hours.	3 Have a drink ready for him when he gets home from work. Have one for yourself too, and maybe you'll have a tantalizing Tuesday night together. You service him with the drink; he'll service you later in bed!	4 Hump Day! Need I say more?	5 Cook him a great steak the manly way (see box).	6 Make it a Freaky Friday. Walk into the room naked with a black leather riding crop in your hand and let the fun begin.	7 Do his laundry . . . in your lingerie and heels!
8 Serve him a Bloody Mary for "breakfast" in bed.	9 Mondays suck. Wink-Wink.	10 Surprise him at work with lunch, dressed to the nines.	11 Hump Day! No explanation necessary.	12 Hop into the morning shower with him.	13 Let him choose the movie to see on date night.	14 Play his video games with him.
15 Let him cheat on you . . . with you. Wear a sassy wig or colored contacts or dress in a fantasy costume (Princess Leia and Wonder Woman are sure to please).	16 Ask him how his day was and really listen. If he doesn't want to talk, let it go.	17 Watch an X-rated video together.	18 Hump Day! You know what to do.	19 Let him know you're proud of him. Send him an email with 10 reasons you're happy to be his girlfriend. (Make it about him and not about what he does for you!)	20 Give him some space. Go rock the town with the girls.	21 Treat him to a striptease.

22 Wake up late and then spend the entire afternoon in bed with him.	**23** Find an exciting new restaurant to try out together.	**24** "Two for Tuesday." Have sex twice today.	**25** Hump Day! Enough said.	**26** Forget the diet and order in pizza and buffalo wings for a night of TV.	**27** Make it Fellatio Friday.	**28** Don't tell him to "turn it down" while he's practicing guitar.

29 Watch the game WITH him for once.

30 Don't have a "Blue Monday" because you've worked your tail off all month for your man. Get that riding crop back out, snap it on his behind, and tell him in your best dominatrix voice: "Next month, it's MY turn!"

Gotha Stewart's T-Boner Recipe

- Buy a large T-bone steak (size matters).
- Lightly cover the meat with salt and pepper and several squirts of Worcestershire sauce. Add cayenne pepper for extra spice. Men like it hot and spicy!
- Brush oil on the grill so the meat doesn't stick.
- Cook the steak on each side to his desired doneness. Most men like it on the rare side, so make sure to keep an eye on that steak and don't overcook it.
- Serve with French fries and a garlic mayonnaise dipping sauce. (For the dipping sauce, simply add some garlic salt to mayonnaise.)

INDIVIDUALITY

By British singer-songwriter Imogen Heap

"It's important to express yourself in your clothing because you never know who you are going to meet that day or what will happen. You should dress as if you are going to meet the man of your dreams that day. If you want to be seen by others as you see yourself, your clothing should represent that. You are a walking advertisement for yourself. And people can't help but make certain judgments upon meeting you, so you want to make sure they are seeing *you* on that first impression. And you are more likely to attract people who are like you if you are always dressing like the individual you are. I like to meet interesting and quirky people, so that is how I dress because that is who I am.

You can't worry about what others say about you or about what you wear. You can't be afraid to do what you want or to be different than others. I just went for it at the Grammys in 2007. I had never been to the Grammys before, let alone be nominated, and I was just over the moon. I assumed since it was a music event, people would dress up crazy and it would be like a rock and roll concert. So, I thought, "Okay. Let's have some fun with this."

Since I'm British and from "across the pond," I wanted to have a theme of pond life. The designer, Pinar Eris, came up with this fabulous black skirt with lily pads on it, and I had wanted my hair really big so I said, "Let's put some grass and twigs in it." I had my white gloves and parasol. Of course, I needed a friend to come with me, so I brought a toy frog named Gary the Grammy frog. It was a total pond theme.

I loved my outfit, and it put me in a good mood for the whole of the Grammys. It made me happy, and afterward, when the bad press came out, to be honest, I didn't really care. I was being me, and I had a blast and I met a lot of interesting people because of it. And to me, that was all that mattered.

INFIDELITY PACTS

By Terri Nunn

"First things first: Most guys aren't going to fuck up a good thing if it's good. It's important to know this and take some responsibility if love goes south. It's important to make him feel amazing in bed. Every time you fuck him, tell him how gorgeous he is and how you've thought about something he did to you for days . . . it's foreplay!

There's no question you're going to be attracted to others during your main relationship. What works for me and my man is an agreement we have: If either one of us just can't stand it and we just have to have someone else we've met, then we can . . . once. We have to tell each other first and get the other's okay too. This agreement has made us both feel like our marriage isn't a cage. Neither one of us has acted on it yet. In almost ten years of togetherness, I've been close a couple of times but didn't follow through, and I don't regret it. I know this wouldn't work for everyone, but it does for us.

The important thing is making an agreement of some kind. If there isn't one, infidelity is more likely to happen. When a man cheated on me, the hardest part was the trust he betrayed. That old saying is true: Trust is hard to get and even harder to get back. If there are continuous absences, you might look into some of the excuses he's given. Some cheating men exhibit more jealousy all of a sudden—more than usual. So that's also a red flag.

Once it's found out, the only thing that will save the relationship—if you still want it—is recommitting to an agreement together, whatever works for the both of you. If it's broken again, now there's a pattern. This guy might not be trustworthy. Without trust, there's no relationship. It's time for counseling if you still want to be in this.

INSPIRATION

By fashion designer Christian Joy, who dresses Karen O. of the Yeah Yeah Yeahs

"Ziggy Stardust is a huge inspiration for me. I think about David Bowie costumes and makeup for Ziggy Stardust each time I create a costume for Karen O. He had this look of being not from this planet, an androgynous alien. I find that exceptionally intriguing. It gives people something exciting to look at and to think about. I don't understand why more rock stars don't give themselves a look.

But John Waters is my biggest inspiration. I love his films. I love how absurd they always are. I was inspired by hearing that he taught himself how to make films. I taught myself fashion design. There is a sort of playfulness that comes out of learning as you go. You have no guidelines to adhere to, and I think it gives you more of an opportunity to take it to different levels. You have to cover your mistakes, so you come up with lots of ideas to do so, and it in turn makes the piece special.

Oddly enough, though, it was not so much one of his films, even though I am often excitedly inspired by them, but a photograph in a fashion magazine that he took that really has kept me thinking over the years. It was a photo of a giant tiger shrimp in a shoe, and my first reaction was "What? I don't get it. That's stupid." Things are always kind of stupid when you don't understand them. I saw the photo before I was making Karen's costumes or even doing fashion design. Then I started to make Karen's costumes, and suddenly that image of the shrimp in the shoe popped into my head again and I realized how really great and funny it was and from there the shrimp sort of became this really hilarious prop-esque thing for me. I actually made Karen a dress with a giant stuffed shrimp that hung like a stole around her neck. It was really funny. Karen ripped it apart with her teeth at a show in London and spit it in the audience. That was the best thing that could have ever happened to that shrimp. The outfit just kept on giving.

Later, the shrimp photo came full circle for me when I saw a documentary on John Waters. In it he talks about "shrimping," which is a type of foot fetish for people who like to suck toes. Eight years later, I finally figured that photo out!

Yoko Ono is another inspiration. I read something about a piece of art that she made that was meant to represent the '60s. And then, in the '80s, she changed the piece by pouring gold over it. I like the idea of a piece evolving or even being useful. That's why it doesn't really bother me to see Karen destroy a costume. I feel like she's adding to it instead of taking away. She's causing it to evolve and giving it a whole new spirit.

I love reading about the New York punk scene. I love the whole DIY aspect of it. The whole spirit of figuring: "If that guy can do it, then so can I." For me, it's never really been about the music. It's always been about the characters involved and how they made it work—bands like the Ramones or the New York Dolls. I like those bands, but I'm more interested in the fact that they just went for it.

My mom is another very, very big inspiration. She was a really DIY mom. There were six kids in our family and we didn't have much money, but she was always coming up with ideas to keep us fed and clothed. One time, she said that she and my dad were at a buffet-style restaurant and my dad left a rather large sausage on his plate.

She thought to herself, "I could make a soup out of that." So she put the sausage in her purse and brought it home. My mom always had a great sense of humor about this sort of thing, which has influenced me.

I am immensely inspired by watching Karen perform. Even just being her friend inspires me. She has a great sense of humor onstage, and she's not worried whether or not her dress is on straight or her lipstick is smeared. She's just fully going for it and it's super attractive, especially to kids who are very often going through that awkward stage of growing up. She makes you feel good and, in a way, relieved.

I guess the style I've created for Karen has really sort of run the gamut from DIY punk to dresses like the shrimp dress that was John Waters–inspired to space alien to voodoo skeleton and most recently to a more Goth sort of look. She wears whatever I give her—even the really awful stuff. One time, I made her this dress that I called the "What's Eating Karen O.?" and which she calls the "Baby on an Acid Trip" or "Pizza Dress." It was fairly hideous, but she came out onstage in it and totally rocked it out like she was wearing the most beautiful dress imaginable. The dress was inspired by Japanese artist Yayoi Kusama. I had seen an exhibition by her at the Museum of Modern Art in New York that was a mirrored room filled with stuffed spotted phalluses. And I thought this was a great idea for a dress.

I think Karen O. is the ultimate rock chick because she doesn't give a fuck. She totally 100 percent goes for it. And that is very inspiring.

INTERVENTIONS

Fourteen signs that you need to hold an intervention for your boyfriend:

1 He has been up for three days straight—for the fourth time this month.

2 He only returns your emails between the hours of 2 a.m. and 7 a.m.

3 Every time you go to his house, there's one more electronic device or guitar missing.

4 In the middle of summer, he is wearing a sweater and shivering.

5 He declares anything from a rooftop at a party after midnight. Cautionary examples include "I am the Lizard King" (Jim Morrison) or "I am a Golden God" (Russell Hammond, *Almost Famous*).

6 His apartment always smells like incense, and there are far too many empty pizza boxes lying around for the number of people who live there.

7 He's constantly itching, picking at his skin, or running for a tissue.

8 His teeth start falling out. And he doesn't play hockey!

9 He forgets complete conversations.

10 He hasn't shown up for band practice in days.

11 He totally forgets YOUR name.

12 When you call him on looking like hell, he says, "I'm coming down with a cold," and you notice that he's *always* coming down with a cold.

13 Snot is running down his nose and he doesn't even feel it dripping!

14 He talks about himself in the third person.

If just a few of these situations sound even remotely familiar, it's time to take him to rehab!

TOP SIGNS THAT YOU ARE ABOUT TO WALK INTO YOUR OWN INTERVENTION:

1 You've been told there's a killer party tonight. But when you pull up you see your grandmother's car in the driveway.

2 Everyone in your life has been acting weird around you all day.

3 Even your cat won't look you in the eyes today.

4 You screwed up royally the night before and the people closest to you didn't freak out, pick a fight, or give you shit about it.

TOP 12 REASONS SOBRIETY ROCKS

By Louise Post of Veruca Salt

1 Less falling down onstage

2 No late-night drunk dialing

3 No hangovers or puffy eyes for your photo shoot the next day

4 Less likely to ill-advisedly make out with one (or more) of your bandmates

5 Ability to maintain your dignity and integrity in all situations

6 Less likely to say controversial shit onstage that will follow you around for the next ten years!

7 Recognizing all of the people in last night's cell-phone pics

8 Making bus call because you're not waking up in a strange hotel room across town

9 No throwing up while your drummer holds your hair

10 Fewer embarrassing YouTube posts!!

11 No stress going through customs

12 Being a clean, pristine, rocking machine

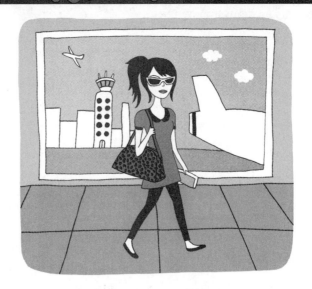

JET-SETTING

A true rock and roll lifestyle always involves a fair amount of traveling. But now that you're a rock chick, you can leave the *traveling* to your aunt Edna—rock stars *jet-set*. It ain't always pretty, but there are ways to glam up your globe-trotting. Here are a few do's and don'ts on how to roll worldwide with a serious air of multi-platinum badassness.

DO

■ Leave your house with some seriously durable luggage. Globe-trotting DJ Paul Oakenfold relies on Tumi. This luggage says two things about a person: I'm rich and I'm indestructible. You could go with designer luggage like Louis Vuitton, but baggage handlers in Bangkok will treat it just the same as a bargain brand no matter who you are. Best to stick to military strength for checked bags and use the more stylish Vivienne Westwood and Betsey Johnson bags for carry-ons.

■ Wear your Marc Jacobs sunglasses from door to door. Not only will it make everyone wonder which fabulous person could be behind them, but it's also just annoying enough to make other passengers assume you couldn't be anyone but a Grammy award–winning recording artist.

■ Bring your own luxury travel pillow, just like Nicole Richie. Duxiana's goose-filled down sleeper with a water-repellent travel case is a good one. The importance of your shut-eye justifies the $100 price tag.

■ Log your frequent flyer miles and try to achieve elite status with airlines. The first people to get upgraded on an oversold flight are those with a high standing in the airline's frequent flyer program. Join them all.

■ Dress to impress. Show up for your flight dressed for a night on the town, not an overnight stay in the emergency room. Swap the sweatpants or yoga pants for ass-hugging suede or leather and cute slip-ons or ballet flats (carry your Dolce & Gabbana heels in your hand luggage to make a graceful exit at your final destination). The gate attendants will notice you and treat you with respect. And remember: A rock chick would never, under any circumstances, be caught dead in Crocs, flip-flops, sneakers, or Birkenstocks.

■ Order up! Rock stars pass the time on long-haul flights by keeping the booze coming . . . and then passing out. Just remember to hydrate with water!

DON'T

■ Pack like you're running away from home. You're going to someplace fabulous, not a shelter. Pack like a pro and you'll never overpack (models often stuff two weeks' worth of clothes into one carry-on!). Some tips: Stuff your boots and shoes with your socks and stockings; a scarf can be used around your neck one day and as a belt the next day, so pack one that can do double duty. Roll your clothes instead of folding them. And always pack a pair of tights, a black cardigan, a pair of skinny pants, a pencil skirt, and black high heels—they go with everything and mix and match well.

CHERRY BOMB

■ Stand in line like cattle at the airline's check-in desk. Don't even bother with the self-serve electronic kiosks, either. The only serving going on here should be that of an airline employee serving you. Drop your luggage at the curbside check-in and snicker at everyone else as you saunter by them on the way to security.

■ If you're stuck in coach, don't fret. Rock stars spend a fair amount of time there too. But under no circumstances should you put up with any of the following: a screaming baby, a toddler kicking the back of your seat, an overweight sloth infringing on your personal space, or anyone behind you whining about you reclining your seat. Ask to be moved immediately. If the flight is full in coach, politely inform the flight attendant that you saw a few empty seats in business class.

■ Whether you're on a plane or a tour bus, or chilling backstage or in your hotel suite, duty almost always calls for the following essentials: Downey Wrinkle Releaser (as if you'd even think about ironing), Purell hand sanitizer, Wet Ones baby wipes, a Tide to Go stain removal stick, an iPod, a few good headbands (it fancies up even the messiest of hairdos), a battery-operated curling iron or Velcro curlers, and (if you need it) Xanax.

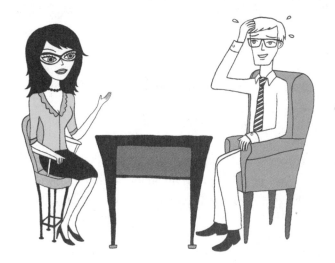

" *There's a better life
and you think about it,
don't you?"*
~DOLLY PARTON, "9 TO 5"

TAKE YOUR JOB AND SHOVE IT!

Good news. You have the skills to get a cooler, more exciting job with really great perks. You're even already doing that job. You're just not doing it for the right company.

Why be an accountant at a company that makes boxes when you can be an accountant at a record label and get free CDs, concert tickets, a sneak peek at rock stars' extravagant expenses all day long? Why work your human resources magic on boring nine to fivers for a company that makes paper when you can help a magazine hire its next Hunter S. Thompson? Need I go on?

Don't expect to be running the show at an exciting new company anytime soon—you might be stuck stuffing envelopes in a cubicle for a while. But trust me, cubicles aren't so bad when you know that at the end of the day your boss could be handing you tickets to a concert, a movie screening, or some cool cocktail party.

HOW TO BREAK INTO THE ENTERTAINMENT INDUSTRY

THE QUICK LIST

■ Be sincerely passionate about the job. Don't just go for it for the perks or prestige. Swag-whores and wannabes won't last long in this highly competitive industry.

■ Know your shit! You shouldn't work in the music business if you don't know what "number one with a bullet" means, and you shouldn't go for a film industry gig if you have no idea what "rose-bud" is.

■ Network your butt off. The entertainment industry is more about who you know than what you know.

■ Be immersed in the scene you want to work in. If it's music, go to shows. If it's film, see every movie you can. If it's TV, you better have a few TiVos in your home.

■ Start a blog about the area of the entertainment industry that you're passionate about.

■ Realize that a job in the music or entertainment industry is not for the faint of heart. If the thought of seeing a band play at midnight leaves you whining about your beauty sleep, don't give up your desk job.

■ Be willing to make little money when you start out and to do crappy jobs for crappy bosses.

■ Have a thick skin. The entertainment industry isn't all hugs and kisses.

■ Just because the entertainment industry might be a tad more laid back than other industries doesn't mean you should try to sleep your way to the top or party your way into the corner office. Reputations are uber-important, and connections are how you get jobs in creative fields. And the entertainment industry is shockingly small—everyone

CARRIE BORZILLO-VRENNA

knows or has heard of everyone. So, sleep with the bossman at one job and it will follow you throughout your entire career.

"HOW I GOT MY COOL CAREER . . ."

Anna Geyer, marketing coordinator and co-promoter of "Girl School" (a weekly night of cool music) at the Viper Room in L.A., says: "In college I knew my passion was music. I don't play any instruments, but I just loved listening to music and going to shows. So even though my major at USC was political science with a cinema minor, I started interning at record labels. First Capitol Records, and then I went to Sony BMG. I had a lot of fun. And then I found an ad on www.enter tainmentcareers.net for an assistant job to the general manager at the Viper Room. I wasn't twenty-one yet; I was twenty. But I applied for it, and I was the first email that the GM got. When he called me in for an interview, he warned me that it was not a sexy job. I came in, and he said, 'When do you want to start?' And I said, 'Right now.' I think being the first to apply had a lot to do with it. Timing and luck have a lot to do with getting jobs in the music industry."

Melissa Renee Hernandez, co-talent buyer and co-promoter of "Girl School" at the Viper Room in L.A., says: "I went to a lot of shows in high school. When I graduated, I found a job at Drive-Thru Records, and they hired me to do PR, which I didn't know a lot about. But I went to a lot of shows and hung out with a lot of bands and people in the industry. I knew [club promoter] Eddy Numbskull when he first started handing out flyers, and DJ Steve Aoki back in the day. I think that had a lot to do with it. I was just an L.A. girl in the music scene, and I got jobs that way (by knowing people and being at the right place at the right time). I started at the Viper Room doing general office assistant work, but because I knew so many L.A. bands I promoted a night of music at 'Indie 103.1 FM' and got all my friends to play. I didn't go to college, but I was streetwise, and I was genuinely, *genuinely* interested in music. I love rock and roll."

Tina Patrick, production coordinator of ABC's *Dancing with the Stars*, says: "Getting recommended for a job makes your job search a lot easier, and the best way to do that is to do each task

CHERRY BOMB

assigned to you at your current position, no matter how small or mundane, to the best of your ability and with a positive attitude. Doing well gives you a good reputation, which is how I was recruited from my online journalism gig to my first job in TV as a writer for MTV News. I landed at my current position at *Dancing with the Stars* in a similar way—a producer I had worked with previously knew the show was staffing up and suggested I apply for it. It all goes back to just doing a great job at all of your jobs because you never know when or how one job will lead you to something even better."

A note from yours truly: Getting here was all about hustling, networking, and being very aggressive. I started out writing for free for my local music fanzines. I landed my first national magazine assignment (the Black Crowes, *Hit Parader*) at age nineteen after I sent the editor my clips and resumé in the form of a mock *Hit Parader* magazine. In college I did two free internships (Columbia Records and Sterling's magazines) and one paid one (*Entertainment Weekly*). I was pretty experienced by the time I got my college degree, but what got me that first job (at *Billboard*) was this: I FedExed my resumé/clips to the editor the day the ad for the job came out, and I followed up immediately with a call. I impressed them with my enthusiasm at the interview, and then I sent an "I'm perfect for this job" follow-up email within hours of the interview.

THE JOB INTERVIEW

■ All in the Mind: Walk into that boss's office with the mind-set that she should be nervous interviewing you, not the other way around.

■ Look Hot: Dress sharper than your boss. Just don't overdo it. For really important interviews, get a blow-out at the salon and a free makeup application at a cosmetics counter at the mall. Leave the short skirts and boob-baring tops at home. Instead, wear a sharp pantsuit (try Nanette Lepore for a sharp, modern, but still rock chick–cool suit) or a pencil skirt and blouse in the summer or a pencil skirt and black turtleneck sweater in the winter.

■ Start Strong: With a firm handshake, look the potential boss in the eye and boldly state, "Hi. I am perfect for this job. I've done this work before and I am not embarrassed to say I'm really good at this job."

■ Be Prepared: Not only should you do your research on the company and your boss, but you should also come in with three concrete reasons why you are qualified for the job. Come with facts and figures and specific achievements from your last position.

■ Avoid Clichés: Instead of saying you're a people person, a hard worker, and eager to please, try these instead: "I've never had problems with bosses or coworkers," "I'm used to working fifty-hour weeks," and "My career is my top priority right now."

■ Take Charge: Don't just sit back and let yourself get grilled; you should be asking some hard questions too—about management style, the company's growth potential, and where THEY see themselves as a company in five years.

■ Negotiate Wisely: Sometimes you need to bluff to get what you want. Let them think your last salary was 15 percent more than it really was so that your starting salary at this job will immediately start out higher than your last. Later, when you go in for a raise, inflate what you want by 5 percent. If you go in asking for a 15 percent raise, they will talk you down to 10 percent. So if you ask for 20 percent, you'll get that 15 percent.

If doing your same job but at a sexier company isn't the complete change you wanted, then maybe it's time to take your skills and see how they apply to a totally new career.

𝕿HE GREAT JOB SWAP

CURRENT JOB	SKILLS USED	NEW JOB
Phone sales	Sexy phone voice, love of headsets	Phone sex operator
Office manager	Good at bossing people around, feeling superior	Dominatrix
Office assistant	Willingness to do demeaning jobs for unthankful people	Celebrity personal assistant
Bathroom attendant at club	Able to listen in on three conversations at once and get people to tip you in the end	Tabloid informant
Babysitter	Ability to deal with loads of shit	Celebrity nanny
UPS loading guy	Can move heavy boxes in a single bound	Roadie
Pharmacist	Access to drugs	Drug dealer to the stars
Travel agent	Has hookups, gets free upgrades	Tour manager
Social worker	Great at giving out advice	Life coach
Clothing store salesperson	Loves to shop and dress others up	Celebrity stylist
Stripper	Great dance skills	Duh, backup dancer for a pop star!
Superfan	Knows everything about their favorite band	Favorite band's official webmaster (Case in point: Trent Reznor hired a superfan to run his Nine Inch Nails website years ago.)

SOUNDTRACK FOR CHANGING JOBS

1. Dolly Parton, "9 to 5"

2. Donna Summer, "She Works Hard for the Money"

3. The Bangles, "Manic Monday"

4. Shonen Knife, "Lazybone"

5. Johnny Paycheck, "Take This Job and Shove It"

6. The Beatles, "A Hard Day's Night"

7. Loverboy, "Workin' for the Weekend"

8. Dire Straits, "Money for Nothing"

9. Todd Rundgren, "Bang the Drum All Day"

BETSEY JOHNSON

What Makes Betsey Johnson Rock?

etsey Johnson is like the superhero of fashion designers. She dresses in Technicolor, cartwheels down the runway, and rocks her multicolored hair like a true rock star.

Johnson (born August 10, 1942, in Wethersfield, Connecticut) is known for her girlie and whimsical designs and for her bold use of colors and prints, which often pair hot pink, lime green, and turquoise. The result is always fun, wild, eccentric, and screams Girl Power, but with an edge.

The designer, who is a strong advocate in the fight against breast cancer after her bout with the disease in 1999, was part of Andy Warhol's scene in New York in the '60s and the whole "Youthquake" fashion, music, and art movement. Warhol's muse, Edie Sedgwick, was her house model, and she also dressed such legendary models as Twiggy and Verushka in their heydays.

Johnson's rock cred goes back to this time, as well as when she dressed art-rock band the Velvet Underground both onstage and off, and ended up marrying (and later divorcing) one of the group's founding members, John Cale. And in the early '70s, she worked for the rock and roll clothing label Alley Cat.

Over the years, she's shown that fashion can be fun by creating pink tutus, hippie chick florals, silver micro-minis, prom-inspired dresses, and clothing and accessories adorned with everything from hearts and oversized lips to cherries and spiders. Her tiered ruffled dresses with tight bustier tops make perfect birthday party dresses for birthday girls of all ages.

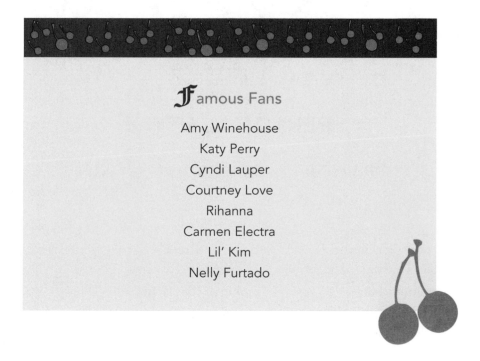

𝔉amous Fans

Amy Winehouse

Katy Perry

Cyndi Lauper

Courtney Love

Rihanna

Carmen Electra

Lil' Kim

Nelly Furtado

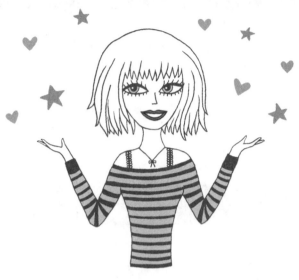

PERSONAL STYLE

By fashion designer Betsey Johnson

CARRIE BORZILLO-VRENNA

"Personal style comes from deep down. You have to want to experiment. You have to want to play around with it. You have to want to give it a try. If you don't really want to, it's not going to look right no matter what you do because your heart and soul ain't in it.

For inspiration, it's okay to find someone who you identify with. Someone in a music video or on a reality television show. You find some girls and guys you identify with because of their style, their look, or their attitude. You try to figure out what it is that makes it work. I think it's all out there to be inspired by, copied, lifted, or whatever you want to do with it. But you have to do it your own way or you'll look like a copy. It's not like you're an uptown girl but you're gonna copy a downtown girl from a magazine and it's gonna work. You have to love it. Take Amy Winehouse—I love the way she looks. I love her hair. I love her makeup. I love her style. I love her tattoos. I love her dresses. I'm so happy that she wears my dresses! But there is a talent to what she does. I just sell a dress. It's only when the girl puts it on that she makes it something of her own. And what she makes it into, or what she doesn't make it into, is really based on what she's about deep down.

You don't learn anything without giving it a try. The only guarantee of trying something new is that you are going to fail. But you have to take a chance, and you've got to lose to win.

You can't really tell how something looks on you. Give your new getup a try for your girlfriends or boyfriends—someone who will give you an honest opinion. Have play dates with girlfriends. Ask them to bring all different types of clothes—conservative, rock and roll, uptown shopping ladies, 8th Street punk, casual girls, the sexpot girl—all of it. And try on outfits for each other. Set it up like an *American Idol* type of thing where you are really going to criticize the outfit and you're really going to try to help the friend make the outfit into what they want to be. Take Poloraids of the outfits, because you can see it differently on the photo than you do with your naked eye. That is what we do when we're getting ready for fashion shows. You're able to play around with fashion without spending money.

What kept me in this industry is that I represented something new, something different, that you couldn't get anywhere else but with me. My courage to do that came from my love for something wacko, something a little different, a little shorter, a little bolder, a little tighter, a little ballerin-y. That is what kept me alive in the business—the fact that I did bring something new.

Change is good. When it works, it feels like "Wow. I've come alive!" I believe in [the 1957 Joanne Woodward movie about a girl with multiple personalities] *The Three Faces of Eve.* I do believe there are all really important personalities inside of all of us, and they should all have a shot at coming out. And they make you feel different. I think how you look totally influences how you feel.

As people get older, I guarantee everyone will end up with a look of their own because it's an accumulation of their life.

"JUST FRIENDS"

We women are pretty intuitive, but even the sharpest chick can sometimes be a little slow on the uptake when she wants to believe something that isn't necessarily true. I'm talking about that guy you've been palling around with. The one you think you might be dating but aren't really sure if he views you as just a friend or as a potential paramour. Here's a list of possible wake-up calls that might indicate that he's already relegated you into that dreaded friend zone:

① He interrupts a deep conversation you're having with him—the kind where your eyes are locked and you think you're really connecting—to ask you if you saw the rack on the hottie who just sauntered by.

② You ask him if you look fat in your new outfit, and he says, "Yes, but not as fat as the dress you wore to the concert last Friday."

③ He recounts intimate tales from past sexual escapades to you.

④ He asks what you'd like to drink and then asks if you have $20 to cover the cost.

⑤ You invite him up for a drink and he declines for ANY reason—even food poisoning.

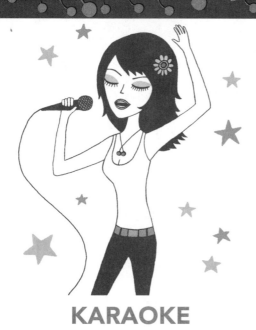

KARAOKE

A great way to get over a fear of public speaking is to get up in front of a crowd at a karaoke bar where nobody knows you and rock out to a few songs. You don't have to sing well, you just need to do your thing with flair and confidence. Don't be nervous. Put on a high-energy show, shake your booty, and have fun with it. Belting out any of these strong rock chick songs—or, for that matter, any song mentioned in this book—will help you unleash the strong, confident, bold woman you have in you. If you can pull this off, then giving a presentation in a meeting or asking for a raise should be a piece of cake!

1 Joan Jett & the Blackhearts, "I Love Rock 'N Roll"

2 Gwen Stefani, "Hollaback Girl"

3 Aretha Franklin, "Respect"

4 Avril Lavigne, "Complicated"

5 Madonna, "Like a Virgin"

6 Kelly Clarkson, "Since U Been Gone"

CHERRY BOMB

7 Helen Reddy, "I Am Woman"

8 The Go-Go's, "We Got the Beat"

9 The Black Eyed Peas, "My Humps"

10 Kelis, "Milkshake"

11 Shakira, "Hips Don't Lie"

12 No Doubt, "Just a Girl"

13 The Weather Girls, "It's Raining Men"

14 Britney Spears, "Oops! . . . I Did It Again"

15 Beyoncé, "Crazy in Love"

16 Tina Turner, "Proud Mary"

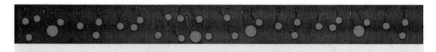

Best Karaoke Duets

Elton John & Kiki Dee, "Don't Go Breaking My Heart"
Olivia Newton-John & John Travolta,
"Summer Nights" from *Grease*
Sonny & Cher, "I Got You Babe"

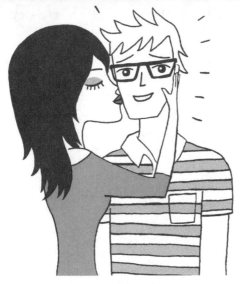

KARMA

Karma is a concept prevalent in Buddhism and Hinduism that essentially states that you get what you deserve. (It's also the title of a cool song by Alicia Keys.) Okay, that's not the technical *Webster's* dictionary definition of it, but basically karma promotes the idea that what you put out there in the world will come back to you. If you put out negativity, you'll get negativity back. If you put out peace, love, and understanding, then you'll get all that gooey stuff back. And, yes, this includes what you may or may not have done in previous lives as well.

So, if you're having a run of bad luck, maybe you just have some ancient bad karma you need to work on overcoming. John Lennon probably didn't have these following tips in mind when he wrote the song "Instant Karma," but they might just help you shine on like the moon and the stars and the sun. So go ahead and try these selfless nice acts to get a dose of Instant Karma coming your way soon.

1 Kiss a geek.

2 Let your mother fix you up on a blind date.

CHERRY BOMB

3 Leave a 25 percent tip at your local mom-and-pop diner.

4 Buy a stranger a beer.

5 Buy the "Instant Karma: The Amnesty International Campaign to Save Darfur" CD at www.instantkarma.org. The double CD features songs by such rockin' chicks as Christina Aguilera, Corinne Bailey Rae, and Regina Spektor, as well as Black Eyed Peas, Green Day, U2, R.E.M., Aerosmith, Lenny Kravitz, and others.

6 Do some volunteer work. (Yours truly volunteers at the Wildlife Waystation, www.wildlifewaystation.org.)

7 Let someone else have the right of way.

8 Say "I'm sorry" . . . and mean it.

9 Stop and listen to what that lady with the petition outside the grocery store has to say.

10 Compliment a female stranger; a simple "Great hair!" will do.

KISS, KEEP, OR KICK OUT?

Girls just wanna have fun, right? But sometimes we need to evaluate just what kind of fun we're after on any given night out. For instance, sometimes the guy we thought was cute from across the club gets closer and blows it in the first ten seconds. And sometimes we meet that guy and go home dreaming that he's "the one." Here are some guidelines to help you figure out—right then and there—if he's good for a smooch or two, a possible keeper, or someone you need to kick to the curb immediately and carry on partying with your girlfriends.

	KISS	KEEP	KICK OUT
He's superhot.	✓		
He's supersexy.	✓		
You're superdrunk.	✓		
It's been a while since you got any.	✓		
He smells good.	✓		
He's an A-lister and someone to write home about.	✓		

	KISS	KEEP	KICK OUT
He's a gentleman.		✓	
He's attentive.		✓	
He asks you questions about yourself.		✓	
He doesn't ignore your friends . . . but he's not too friendly with them, either.		✓	
He makes you feel good.		✓	
He asks for your number and tells you he'd like to take you out on a date.		✓	
He doesn't try to nail you that night.		✓	
His shirt is unbuttoned Jesse Metcalfe–style or he's sweating like a pig Brandon Davis–style.			✓
He's drinking a girlie cocktail.			✓
You smell his cologne from across the room.			✓
He's got an orange fake-tan.			✓
His friends look like losers.			✓
He unloads a cheesy pickup line on you.			✓

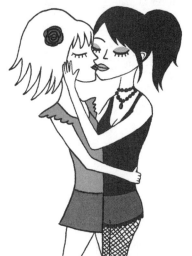

I was open about it [bisexuality] because I wanted people to know that I had been with a woman. I spoke about it because I'd discovered something wonderful and I thought people should know my experience was very real, very normal."

~ANGELINA JOLIE *(ELLE)*

LESBIAN, BISEXUAL, OR BI-CURIOUS? QUIZ

So, you were enjoying girls' night out and oops, your tongue ended up in some chick's mouth. Okay, you kissed a girl. And you liked it. Now you're questioning who you are. Don't fret. I know big questions of identity can't be answered with a little quiz, but they're fun to take and might shed a *little* light on your preferences. So take this one and see if it helps you on the road to figuring out if you're a lesbian, bisexual, or just a little bi-curious, like most naughty girls are.

1 After you kiss a girl during a drunken night out, you . . .

a. freak out when you get home but want to do it again.

b. text her the second you get home and ask her out on a real date.

c. have an erotic dream about her that night and send her flowers in the morning.

2 You have fantasized about . . .

   a. kissing Madonna.

   b. a threesome with Madonna and Guy Ritchie.

   c. going down on Madonna.

3 Your favorite of these three songs is . . .

   a. "I Kissed a Girl" by Jill Sobule.

   b. "Girls & Boys" by Blur.

   c. any song by Peaches.

4 You totally understand how Angelina Jolie or Anne Heche have each been in both lesbian relationships and heterosexual relationships.

   a. Eh. Sort of. Maybe. I guess.

   b. Sure. Why not? Variety is the spice of life.

   c. No way! Pick a team!

5 Which rock star has rocked the androgynous look the best?

   a. Annie Lennox

   b. David Bowie

   c. Grace Jones

6 Your favorite female singer is . . .

   a. Gwen Stefani.

   b. the Sounds' Maja Ivarsson.

   c. the Gossip's Beth Ditto.

7 Your favorite magazine is . . .

   a. the Victoria's Secret catalogue. You like to look at pretty girls.

   b. *Curve*, *Bitch*, and *Diva*. The articles rock.

   c. *Lesbian Life*. You have a lifetime subscription.

8 The sexiest animated/cartoon gal to you is . . .

a. Jessica Rabbit of *Who Framed Roger Rabbit?*

b. Natasha Fatale of *Rocky and His Friends* and *Boris and Natasha: The Movie.*

c. Velma Dinkley of *Scooby-Doo.*

9 You'd most like to get your ass kicked by . . .

a. Lara Croft: Tomb Raider.

b. Frida Kahlo.

c. Joan of Arc.

10 Your cat's name is . . .

a. anything girlie with three or more syllables—Priscilla, Angelina, Jennifer.

b. Sappho.

c. Muffy.

THE ANSWERS COME IN THE FORM OF ENLIGHTENING SONGS AND QUOTATIONS.

IF YOU CHOOSE MOSTLY AS: You dig girls who are boys who like boys to be girls who do girls like they're boys. Confused by that? Don't worry, you're just bi-curious.

IF YOU CHOSE MOSTLY BS: Rodney Dangerfield once said, "Bisexuality immediately doubles your chances for a date on Saturday night." That's good news for you. Better dust off those dancing shoes.

IF YOU CHOSE MOSTLY CS: What else could I say, everyone is gay. Nirvana might have sung that tune in "All Apologies," but no apology is needed if you racked up a lot of Cs. Now go set that season pass for *The L Word.*

CHERRY BOMB

GIRL CRUSH CONFESSIONAL

" ['Mystery Girl'] wasn't about a particular girl. When I first started writing songs, the subject, the person I was singing about or to would be a girl. But there are two types of girls I get crushes on. One is the sort of girl who's really got it together and who has a sort of boyish look and who's really got it going on. And then the other is the blond cheerleader-type who has like a lip ring or something like that but yet is still just clueless. . . . All of my sex dreams are of a same-sex or homoerotic nature. I think those fantasies are because I like playing with gender roles and images. "

~THE YEAH YEAH YEAHS' KAREN O. (*THE ADVOCATE*)

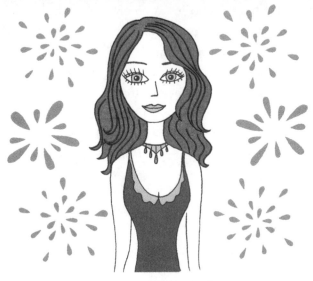

LIFE ADVICE

By singer-songwriter Tori Amos

THREE THINGS I LIVE BY

1 *Discipline:* You can have all the ideas that a person can possibly come up with in a day, but unless you know how to focus your energies and discipline your mind, you will never be able to manifest these ideas. Part of being disciplined is being able to manage your time. In a single day your ideas can dissipate if you spend more time on texting, phoning, or emailing than you do on developing these potential expressions. Being talented is not enough. Wanting success is not enough. Being able to tell your friends and family and everyone else "Now is not a good time, I'm working" is what discipline is about. Those people who really respect what you are doing won't give you a hard time. Another side of discipline is if someone does give you a hard time because you're not in constant contact, you don't bite the big cherry, desert your work, or blow your whole day just to appease a persistent friend.

2 *Recharging:* I have found it extremely important to recharge my body and my mind quite frequently. This does not mean shopping. That's a quick rush, instant gratification, and it doesn't last long. When I go out into nature, I find that I'm able to unload old patterns that don't work for me anymore. Whether that's spending time by the sea or spending time outside of the city in the desert, in the countryside, just anywhere away from parasitic energies. I have found this to be a key component in being able to stay grounded when you get back into the city and into the bustle.

3 *Keeping my creative source as my center:* When we wake up in the morning, we can choose to either "plug in" to the creative source or "plug in" to a chaotic force. If you don't consciously choose this, then you will be drawn into chaos before lunch and you'll have no idea how you got there. Energy follows intention. I wake up, I take the ten minutes it takes—in the shower, putting on makeup, before I go out—to set my intentions, what I will and won't accept energy-wise. There is not one way that is the right way to do this. But if you are aligned with a creative source, then it's very hard to seduce you into destructive conversations, arguments, and reactions. Once you step into that, the unraveling begins. By the time you come home you wonder how in the world your circuits could be so fried in less than twenty-four hours.

A bonus one for the road: When you come up for air . . . come up laughing.

> "Marriage is a great institution, but
> I'm not ready for an institution."
>
> ~MAE WEST

MARRIAGE

A solid, long-lasting, successful marriage for creative couples comes down to agreeing on three little things: sex, drugs, and rock and roll.

SEX: If one person is adventurous and is up for anything (whips, chains, whatever) anytime and the other partner is perfectly satisfied with missionary position once a week, it's probably not a good match. Your adventure level and libido need to be in sync. Likewise, if one views children as the worst possible outcome of sex and the other is already naming their babies, get out now!

DRUGS: One teetotaler and one lush (alcohol's a drug, right?) equal two guaranteed broken hearts down the road.

ROCK AND ROLL: The biggest deal-breaker of all—musical tastes. You could both be into country, rap, or good ol' fashioned rock and roll and live happily ever after, but if a couple is at the opposite ends of the musical spectrum, they'll both be singing the blues in no time.

CHERRY BOMB

THE BRIDE WORE . . . WHAT?

BLACK: Yours truly (Les Habitudes corset and Eavis & Brown skirt)

BLACK: Sarah Jessica Parker

PURPLE: Dita Von Teese (Vivienne Westwood)

GREEN: Kelis (Matthew Williamson)

PINK AND WHITE: Gwen Stefani (John Galliano)

PINK: Mariska Hargitay (Carolina Herrera)

IVORY WITH BLACK SASH: Pink (Monique Lhuillier)

WHITE WITH BLACK SASH AND BLACK NET HAT: Shanna Moakler (Monique Lhuillier)

Dare to be a different bride.

ALEXANDER MCQUEEN

What Makes Alexander McQueen Rock?

R ock and roll has always been daring, adventurous, and dangerous, and that is just what British designer Alexander McQueen's designs represent.

Out of all the designers who music peeps and creative types like the most, McQueen (born March 17, 1969, in London, England) is the most avant-garde and most often misunderstood by the general population.

McQueen, the son of a London taxi driver, has raised eyebrows with runway shows featuring a double amputee model with elaborately carved wooden legs, a robot that sprayed black and yellow ink on a model in a white dress, a hat adorned with mini German warplanes, low-cut pants called the "Bumster," which showed ass-crack cleavage, and women dressed as clowns on a runway made to look like a vintage carousel.

McQueen was once asked who he designs for. His answer? "A strong, independent woman who loves and lives fearless in equal measure." One of the most fearless McQueen wearers is Gwyneth

Paltrow, who is married to Coldplay singer Chris Martin. The A-lister famously wore the designer's Goth-inspired gown with a see-through top to the 2002 Oscars, causing her mainstream movie peers and the fashion police to debate her racy choice.

More recently, fashionista Mary Kate Olsen sported his black-and-white skull scarf ($220), and country singer Leann Rimes regularly totes around his brown patent leather Elvie bag ($1,495). Rimes has said of the accessory, "I love my bag. It livens up any outfit and makes it more rock and roll." Yes, indeed.

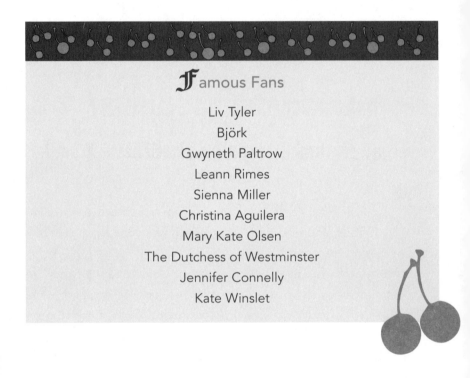

Famous Fans

Liv Tyler
Björk
Gwyneth Paltrow
Leann Rimes
Sienna Miller
Christina Aguilera
Mary Kate Olsen
The Dutchess of Westminster
Jennifer Connelly
Kate Winslet

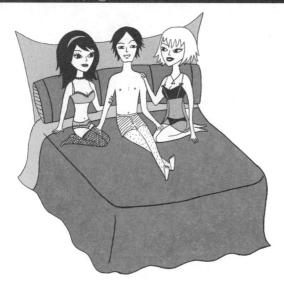

MÉNAGE À TROIS
By adult film star Tera Patrick

"Every single guy wants a threesome. It's all about indulging and living out a fantasy. If you are going to do anything extracurricular like this, you need to make sure that you are in control and that you set boundaries. You should be the main girl, and you can dictate what the other girl can and cannot do with your man. So, you need to talk to both of them ahead of time and set up those boundaries. You need to tell them what you are comfortable with and what you aren't. If you set those rules, no one will get hurt. Choose the girl wisely—and *you* should be the one to pick her. I don't recommend having a threesome with a friend, because it will ruin the friendship and you don't want that memory burned into your brain. And, since it's all about fantasy, you don't want to keep in touch with her after. If she's willing to play by your rules, you may be more inclined to do it again. You just need to say to her, "Hey. I'm willing to share my man with you, but this is what it's all about, and if you don't go along with the rules, I'm going to kick your ass!"

CHERRY BOMB

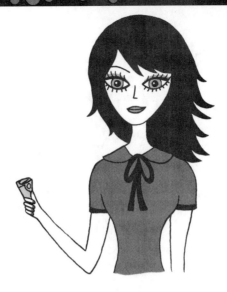

MONEY

How to Get "Back in Black"

Sure, AC/DC was not thinking of personal finances when they wrote their classic rock song, but it's my inspiration when I'm balancing my checkbook.

Being ultra-responsible about money doesn't sound very daring and edgy and dangerous, but it's really the foundation of a, well, daring and edgy and dangerously fun lifestyle. It's hard to live life like a rock star on a bank account more akin to a starving actor. And a truly cool chick doesn't rely on a man to buy her pretty things . . . or pay her rent! Nope, that's not us.

Rockin' cool looks by Jean-Paul Gaultier or Vivienne Westwood takes money and sometimes puts us in the red like the bottoms of our Christian Louboutin shoes. I've been there, and everything on the following list has worked to help me get out of a fat five-figure credit card debt and back in black in no time.

Some of these suggestions might sound inconsequential, but trust me, they add up.

INCREASE YOUR INCOME (DUH!)

❶ Ask your boss for a raise. Before you scoff, "Oh! Why didn't I think of that?" you would be amazed at how many people don't think this is a viable option. Don't wait for your yearly review to get that teeny-weeny cost-of-living raise. Start kicking butt at work more than ever; after a month of truly going above and beyond your job responsibilities, go to your boss with a list of at least five reasons why you deserve a raise now, and just ask for one. It's hard for a boss to say no when he or she is presented with facts and figures and a solid reason why you should get what you're asking for.

❷ Take on some consulting work as a second job. Let's say you're a CPA at your day job. Offer up your services on the side to your friends by doing their taxes. Or, if you work at a clothing store, put out an ad for your "styling" services. If your resumé looks awesome, offer up resumé writing services to pals or post an ad on craigslist. Are you a good organizer? Get paid to organize people's closets, drawers, or homes. Almost any job or skill can be turned into extra freelance money.

❸ Sell your stuff on eBay or have a yard sale. It's amazing how much potential cash you have hanging around your home in the form of old clothes, outdated jewelry, and CDs you've already put into your iPod. Every little bit counts. Sell your crap!

❹ Become a housesitter and/or petsitter for your friends and colleagues when they go away.

CUT DOWN ON YOUR BILLS AND EXPENSES

❶ Call your credit card company and ask for a lower rate. If you've paid your bills on time and been a cardholder for a decent amount of time, they will not want to lose your business.

❷ If you haven't paid your bills on time and don't have good credit, talk to your bank about consolidating any credit card debt or outstanding loans.

CHERRY BOMB

3 Only send your clothes to the dry cleaner if you really, truly have to. Most garments will do just fine with the Dryel sheets that you can buy at the grocery store. I have personally used them on Marc Jacobs tops, Miss Sixty hot pants, and even on a Vivienne Westwood skirt.

4 Take a good, hard look at all of your household bills—phone, cable, insurance, etc.—and shop around for better rates. If you're a home owner, consolidating your home owner's, earthquake or flood, and automobile insurance into one policy with one company can save you money. Get rid of your home phone line and do what the cool kids are doing—have just your cell phone. Try to consolidate your Internet/cable/phone plans.

5 Cancel your magazine and newspaper subscriptions and read your weeklies at work, at the doctor's office, or online.

6 Prescription meds: Ask your doctor if there is a cheaper medicine for whatever ails you. Why spend more on Ambien for sleeping problems when Tylenol PM or Advil PM might surprise you by working just as well?

7 Cancel the housecleaner and use some elbow grease to clean your place. Added bonus: Housework is a good workout, especially for your arms.

8 Stop getting professional manicures and pedicures. Buy a cheap kit and do it yourself at home. Make it more fun by having a spa night with your girlfriends.

9 Likewise, the hair salon can cost a fortune. Until you're back on your pretty pedicured feet financially, have a "Dye & Drink" hairdying party at your house with your girlfriends using over-the-counter products. If Garnier is good enough for Sarah Jessica Parker and L'Oréal's Féria is good enough for Milla Jovovich, it's good enough for anyone. My favorite? Special Effects' rockin' red called Cherry Bomb, of course!

SPEND MORE WISELY

1 Stop clothes shopping. If you want something "new" to wear, dye your lighter clothes another color with Rit fabric dye and they will feel like new. Also, lean on your friends—borrow clothes, shoes, and accessories from your same-size pals!

2 If you must shop, go to thrift stores, the Salvation Army, Goodwill, or consignment shops and dig for treasures.

3 Stop buying top-shelf liquor! A Stoli or Absolut and tonic gets the job done just as well as the more expensive Grey Goose– or Belvedere-based drink.

4 Think before you buy premade meals, sandwiches, and salads at the grocery store, and before you head out to dine at a restaurant. A loaf of bread, a head of lettuce, a bag of carrots, and some pasta and sauce will feed you for a week for less money.

5 Cancel your gym membership and hit the pavement for a jog instead. If jogging is not your thing, it's easy to set up a small home gym even in the tiniest of apartments. Get a few free weights, a mini trampoline, a yoga mat, and some exercise DVDs. Hell, if your cable system has FitTV, like mine does, you don't even need the videos. It's a 24-hour fitness channel with tons of workouts.

6 Kick your expensive coffee habit. Drink your coffee for free at the office or buy a pound of beans for your home and invest in a cheap coffeemaker and a travel mug.

7 Stop getting a spray tan. Jergen's "Natural Glow Daily Moisturizer" is less expensive and looks more natural. Or go pale!

8 Instead of going to dinner with a friend, go to lunch. It's cheaper, even at the most expensive restaurants.

9 Check out the 99-cent store. They carry some name brands like Scotch tape and Colgate toothpaste. Why pay full price if you can get something for 99 cents?

FUN FACT: Avril Lavigne was caught buying holiday wrapping paper at a 99-cent store in November 2007.

CHERRY BOMB

10 We know you're a girl on the go, but stop hitting random ATMs around town when you're out clubbing. This racks up high ATM fees. Only take cash out of your own bank's ATMs, and try to just take money out once a week. Spend only the cash you take out.

SAVE MORE MONEY

1 Just because you sold those old pair of Levi's on eBay for $20 doesn't mean you can go out and get a $20 manicure. Put the money toward paying off your credit card, loans, or a friend who you owe money to.

2 Have a stylish, old-school ceramic piggy bank to put all of your loose change in. Every six months, roll up those coins and cash them in. Even though CoinStar is convenient, they take a percentage of your change that you can't afford to give away, so wrap those pennies, nickels, and dimes yourself and head to the bank. Remember, every little bit helps.

3 If you don't already have a bank with a fee-free plan, switch to one now. There is no reason to be paying service fees if you don't have to.

If you think the above measures are extreme, remember that you don't need to do everything on this list forever. But if you are in debt, do all of this for at least six months. You'll see how fast the extra cash adds up. Once you're back in black, add in a few things you miss the most (like weekly manicures), but if you feel yourself slipping back into the red, you know what to do!

"Good things happen to those who hustle."
~ANAÏS NIN

NETWORKING 101

There's a difference between networking and schmoozing. Schmoozing normally brings to mind some cheesy, insincere "Hollywood" person who's out to use you for his or her own gain. Networking, however, is making connections with solid people in your desired industry to build up your contacts and hopefully get a cool new job or get on a guest list somewhere. Here's how to do it:

■ Attend as many events and parties in your desired field as possible. If you want to work in the music industry, go to concerts regularly and conferences like South by Southwest in Austin, Texas, every spring, or CMJ in New York in the fall.

■ Introduce yourself to strangers at these events and always exchange business cards. Ask them what they do or how they got into their field. People love talking about their own success. Remember: You don't need a job to have a business card, so go get some made up for yourself already.

■ The day after meeting the person, follow up with a quick email saying it was nice to meet him or her. Don't have their card? Track them down, politely, on MySpace, Facebook, or LinkedIn and follow up through those sites.

■ Flatter them. In your follow-up correspondence, tell them you'd like to pick their brain about what they do and offer to take them to lunch. Then follow up with a "thank you for your time" email. (Note: I said *email*, not *text*.)

■ Don't be a jerk. Never dismiss someone just because they are an intern or an assistant, or you think they're too young or too old to help you get ahead. That low-level employee could be running the company the next day. And don't forget, assistants can really influence their bosses and get things done, so be kind to them and learn from them.

ORGASMS:
THE MIND OVER BODY ORGASM

By Dr. Ava Cadell,
founder of www.loveologyuniversity.com

"Since the brain is the most erotic organ in the body, it should be no surprise that you can think your way to orgasm. Sexual thoughts can activate the brain just like sexual touching does. If you've ever enjoyed looking at porn you'll know what I'm talking about. Visuals of people having sex can automatically trigger your body into a state of arousal, making women wet and giving men erections. If you continue to watch erotica without touching yourself, you could still experience a full-blown orgasm. Even if you're not into porn, you can achieve a mind over body orgasm by tapping into all five of your senses. To begin, wet your genitals with your own saliva or some lubricant, and then, using only your imagination, think about what your lover's tongue would feel like between your legs. What he or she smells like when fully aroused, visualize what they look like naked, imagine touching, kissing, and licking and tasting his or her body. Hear them moaning with plea-

CHERRY BOMB

sure. Become aware of your own feelings as you let your excitement build. The trick here is not to touch yourself, but to let the ebb and flow of your orgasm take you on a mental journey to sexual ecstasy. This can also be fun to do with a partner as a safe sex activity.

PARTYING

R—Rock your look. Dress to impress. If you can, work in a hat, a scarf, some bling, a pimp cup, sunglasses at night, and dark nail polish (it doesn't have to be black—deep purple, ruby, or silver make a rock star–style statement too).

O—Overcome your inhibitions. Dance on that table. Take the mic. Kiss a stranger. Kiss a girl.

C—Cash or credit? Neither! Party on someone else's dime. Rock stars don't pay for a thing.

K—Kick it with a sidekick and make sure your pal is as pimped out as you are. Everyone needs a partner like Snoop Dogg's the Bishop (and his bejeweled pimp cup).

S—Say yes to anything and everything without hesitation—to anything offered to you, to any dare, to jumping in the pool on the roof of a hotel, to any fun change of plans, to any request for "just one more!"

$\mathfrak{T}$—Take extra long in the bathroom at a club, with a girlfriend in the same stall, and walk out with your head held high when the line of ladies snicker at you.

$\mathfrak{A}$—Arrive fashionably late.

$\mathfrak{R}$—Remember, the trick is to be an entertaining drunk, not an annoying drunk. Entertaining Drunk = funny, vivacious, dancing on tables, going with the flow, kicking it up a notch by ordering that fourth round of shots. Annoying Drunk = gushing about anyone to their face, saying "I'm so drunk!" or screaming the phrase "Vegas, baby, Vegas!"

HOW TO FAKE "KEEPING UP"

❶ If your rock star host is insisting you do "just one more" shot but you just don't have it in you, pour yours over your shoulder as his head is cocked back and he's swigging down a shot.

❷ Just Say No: Tell him you have a sinus infection.

❸ Always have a full drink in your hand even if it's just water or Coke. Tell 'em the water is straight vodka or the Coke is whiskey.

SIGNS THAT IT'S TIME TO PUT YOUR PIMP CUP DOWN

❶ You're singing the wrong words at karaoke even though the lyrics are scrolling right in front of your face.

❷ That's you in the corner—passed out and drooling.

❸ That last shot of tequila went down your shirt instead of down the hatch.

❹ You forgot to wax down there, yet you stripped and jumped in that pool anyway.

❺ You threw up . . . twice. (Once is okay, but never let your fellow partiers know that you puked. And if asked, lie!)

❻ Everyone keeps saying "What?!?!" to everything you say.

ROCK STAR DRINKS: WHAT'S "IN" AND WHAT'S "OUT"

In

Absinthe

Jack Daniels (as a shot, on ice, or with Coke)

Jägermeister

Scotch, neat

Vodka with one mixer

Beer

Wine (anything red, but not Merlot—Merlot is for soccer moms!)

Champagne

Energy drinks

Tequila

Snakebite (half Crown Royal and half Coke in a shot glass)

Out

Cosmopolitans

Daiquiris

Mudslides

Sex on the Beach shots

Fuzzy Navels

Margaritas (unless you're in Mexico or at a Mexican restaurant)

White wine (that's for brunch)

CHERRY BOMB

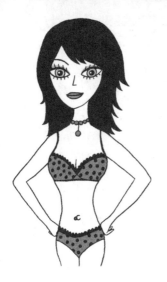
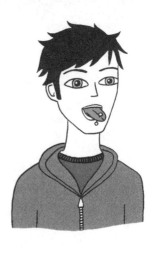

PIERCINGS

By NicoleLee Suicide of SuicideGirls.com

"These days, body piercings aren't just for extremists. Mainstream celebrities like Christina Aguilera, Hayden Panettiere, and Keira Knightly have had piercings on various parts of their bodies over the years. If you're thinking about getting a piercing or have just started dating a guy who has one and you're not quite sure what to make of it, here's a crash course on this form of body modification.

FOR THE LADIES

NAVEL

Pro: You look sexy in a bikini and have more jewelry to shop for.
Con: The yoga pose "cobra" might put you in stitches.

TONGUE

Pro: For him, blow jobs have that "little something extra."
Con: Forget about blowing bubbles with gum.

CLITORAL HOOD

Pro: Wearing tight pants is enough to get you aroused.

Con: Remember to clean your jewelry along with your sheets after sex.

NIPPLE

Pro: Added sensitivity when he gets to second base.

Con: New mommies have to remove them. Simple math: nipple ring + breast-feeding = teething device. Ouch!

𝔉OR THE DUDES

NIPPLE: If your man has a nipple ring, yes, that does mean that he wants you to pull on it.

TONGUE: If he knows what he's doing, cunnilingus will never be the same!

PRINCE ALBERT: This guy is insecure about his length. Seriously.

FRENUM LADDER: These bring a whole new meaning to "ribbed for her pleasure."

STRETCHED EARLOBES: "Do your ears hang low? Do they wobble to and fro?" gets old. Fast.

> *I'm so mean 'cause I cannot get you outta your head,*
> *I'm so angry cause you'd rather MySpace instead,*
> *I can't believe I fell in love with someone that wears more*
>   *makeup than . . .*
> *You're so gay and you don't even like boys."*
>
> **~KATY PERRY, "UR SO GAY"**

QUEER?

We've all been there. *Ooh, he's cute. Hmmm. Is that eyeliner he's wearing? No problem, he's in a band. Wait . . . did he just rent* Brokeback Mountain *for the third time? Well, Okay, it was a good movie. Hmmm. His favorite artist is Cher? Well, she does rock. Well, huh. Hmmm. I don't know. Is my boyfriend gay? Or is he just a sweet, sensitive, in-touch-with-his-feminine-side guy like a lot of creative people are?* If you have to ask yourself too many questions like these, maybe it's time to take a deeper look at your new man. Use this checklist to help you decide if the boy is queer or not.

	STRAIGHT	A LITTLE BIT GIRLIE	GAY
HIS TAKE ON *BROKEBACK MOUNTAIN*	Totally gross	Found it touching	Hoping for *Brokeback Mountain: The After Story*
FAVORITE SPORTS	Football, basketball, baseball, hockey	Soccer, but just to see David Beckham play	Men's wrestling, swimming, figure skating, gymnastics

	STRAIGHT	A LITTLE BIT GIRLIE	GAY
FAVORITE MUSIC	Anything metal, Southern or classic rock, "cock rock"	The Killers, Franz Ferdinand, Blur, the Smiths	Madonna, Donna Summer, Cher, Mika, Scissor Sisters
COMPLI-MENTS	He tells you that you look pretty only on special occasions	He notices every new haircut and new shade of lipstick you wear	He not only compliments your shoes, but he can also tell you the designer who made them, the season they're from, what celebrities have worn them, and on which page of *Us Weekly* he saw them.
FLIRTING	He flirts with pretty girls	He compliments his male friends when they're looking hot	Pretty men flirt with him
MOVES	He tries to get you into bed on the first date	He gets you into bed on date number three and then wants to cuddle all night	You're on date number twelve and no bodily fluids have been exchanged
SEX	He's up for anything except a threesome with a dude	He'd have a threesome if Johnny Depp or Jared Leto were involved	The only door he's up for entering is the back door
GROOMING	He shaves when he has to and is pretty good about keeping the stray nose hairs at bay	He has the same number of grooming products as you	He waxes his body, from eyebrows to toes and everything in between
MAKEUP	He's in a band, so of course he wears makeup! Just like Fall Out Boy's Pete Wentz and everyone in Marilyn Manson	Rockers wear eyeliner, but he adds a little shadow to his lids and gloss to his lips even when he's NOT onstage.	He has way more makeup than you, organized in a three-tiered professional makeup case—the kind the pros use

"It's a bad sign if he's wearing guyliner, if his flat iron is always plugged in, and if you find him wearing your jeans all at the same time. That sums up 'Ur So Gay,'" says Katy Perry.

CHERRY BOMB

159

RED LIPS

By American Idol
and celebrity makeup artist Mezhgan

"Red lipstick works for everyone . . . if they work it. You need to be comfortable with the look in order to wear it well. But the same shade of red lipstick will not work on everyone. You need to base your shade selection on what you plan to do with the rest of your face. For instance, if you are wearing cool tones on your cheeks and eyes, you should pick a red with more red or blue-red tones. If you are wearing warm shades, you should pick a red with a more brown or orange hue. It needs to complement your skin color too.

A good trick of the trade to making red lipstick last all day is to use a concealer and a powder as a base. Then use a lip liner that matches your color, and feather it into your lips before you put on your lipstick. This can be a little drying, so you want to make sure your lips are hydrated so the color will go on smooth and even. A great combo is the Cherry Lip Liner by M.A.C. with my own brand of lip gloss, me by {me}zhgan Kiss Me, in the shade "Sexy Me" over it.

Here are few of the shades that these ladies in red have rocked on the red carpet:

Guerlain Kiss Kiss Lipstick in "Exces de Rouge" (Gwen Stefani)

Christian Dior Rouge Dior in "Celebrity Red" (Christina Aguilera)

M.A.C. Lipstick in "Russian Red" (Dita Von Teese)

Max Factor MAXalicious Glitz in "Vegas Nights" (Carmen Electra)

Smashbox Photo Finish Lipstick in "Ravishing" (Scarlett Johansson)

RESTAURANT RESERVATIONS

Part of living like a rock star is being able to get a table at a hot, hard-to-get-into restaurant. But before you try to become a regular at a super-hoity-toity spot, consider the fact that some of the coolest places for filling your belly aren't always the spots with the highest Zagat rating but historical places with rock and roll history.

For instance, Barney's Beanery in West Hollywood, California, is a great place for burgers and beers and also happens to be the cool restaurant where Janis Joplin partied the night she died. It was also a favorite of Doors' Jim Morrison. Today, the most rockin' dish of all—their "champagne breakfast"—includes a bottle of Dom Perignon and an extra large chili cheese dog with fries for $195 plus tip.

But if it's *living* celebrities you want to see (and potentially rub elbows with, bump into, hit on, or just ogle), then today's five-star restaurants are the places to go . . . if you can get in! Here's how to do just that:

PLAN AHEAD: Don't wait until the last minute to make a dinner date. Plan your night out as far in advance as possible. Some hot spots have waiting lists of two weeks; others are four or five weeks out. Do your research.

TIMING: Pick a less popular time to go. It's easier to get a reservation at the hot restaurant in town if you make it for 6:30 p.m. or 11 p.m. (if they seat diners that late). You won't miss out on any celeb spotting, because your 6:30 p.m. dinner can last until 8:30 p.m. if you eat slowly and order dessert; by the time you're wrapping up, you might spot a famous face walking in. Same goes if you make a reservation for 11 p.m.—as you're coming in, they'll just be getting their party started.

NAME-DROP: If you work at any place even remotely cool, call and pretend you are your own assistant and say you're making a reservation for your boss at so-and-so company. Sometimes just the air of importance makes the difference. Likewise, if you know anyone who knows the chef, work that connection. If you are friends with a food writer, have that pal make the reservation or tell the person taking the reservation that your food writer friend recommended the place.

GO ONLINE: Try www.opentable.com to make your reservation. More than 7,000 high-end restaurants worldwide use this reservation site. They hold a certain number of tables strictly for their online customers, and it's free to use! You should also check out websites and blogs such as Eater to get the behind-the-scenes skinny on new restaurants and how to get on the waiting list for opening night.

GET PERSONAL: Find the email address of the restaurant manager and email him or her directly, saying how much you love their restaurant and are looking to celebrate your birthday, anniversary, promotion, your album going gold, or whatever at their fine dining establishment. A little flattery and a personal touch go a long way.

LADIES WHO LUNCH: If it's really impossible to get that *dinner* reservation you want, why not opt for lunch? Bonus: Lunch is cheaper than dinner. So you'll save some dough and get a great meal at a top restaurant.

CHERRY BOMB

LAST RESORT: If you're stuck in a situation where you need a reservation that night, you can rock it old-school by showing up at the restaurant and greasing the maitre d's palm with a $50 bill. I know this sounds like something straight out of an old movie, but I've seen it done in the twenty-first century and know it works. If you're unsuccessful or don't want to lay out that kind of cash, then ask if you and your friends can eat at the bar. It's often more fun in that area anyway, and bartenders are usually super-cute.

SEX APPEAL

"Personally I think that sexy is keeping yourself mysterious."

~STEVIE NICKS (*FASHION ROCKS*)

"If you're comfortable with yourself, then that's sexy."

~SCARLETT JOHANSSON (L'ORÉAL WEBSITE)

"Sex appeal is 50 percent what you've got and 50 percent what people think you've got."

~SOPHIA LOREN

"My impression is that what they find sexy doesn't make them very interesting or unusual or special. That makes them common."

~SARAH JESSICA PARKER ON MEN WHO PREFER AN AIRBRUSHED WOMAN TO A NATURAL ONE (*ALLURE*, FEBRUARY 2008)

SMOKY ROCK CHICK EYES

Y ou really don't have to be a rock chick like Avril Lavigne, Fergie, or Amy Lee to sport the smoky eye look. Everyone and their mother is rocking this look these days because it's sexy, sultry, and very stylish. And the look isn't just for nighttime anymore. People like the Olsen twins, Kate Moss, and Sienna Miller roam around in the daylight hours sporting a dark, smoky eye.

You can rock this look in any hue, but the blacks, charcoals, grays, purples, and midnight blues work the best for achieving a really sexy, dramatic look. Whatever color palette you use, the key is to have three varying shades. If you're going for the darkest look, you'll want to use some variation of white, gray, and black. The darkest color goes in the crease. The medium shade is for the eyelid. The lightest color is to highlight the area right under the eyebrow.

STEP 1: Using your finger, apply a light layer of your foundation or an eye makeup primer to your eyelids, all the way up to your eyebrows.

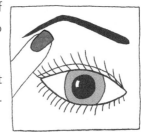

STEP 2: Take your lightest color and swipe it from the top of your eyeball up to the eyebrow.

STEP 3: Apply your medium color to the eyelid from the lashline to the crease.

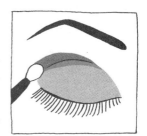

STEP 4: Take your darkest color and apply it to the crease and out to the outermost corner of your eyes, as far out as you are comfortable with going. Start by swiping the color out to the side far enough so it's just even with the end of your eyelid. The key to this step is to use an eye shadow brush that is designed for the crease. It's also best to use a matte shadow in the crease and save the shimmery or glittery shades for highlighting the brow bone or for shining up your lids.

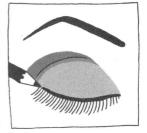

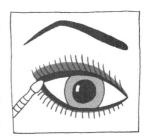

STEP 5: Draw a thin line of black eyeliner close to the lashline.

STEP 6: Line the insides of both your top and bottom lashlines.

STEP 7: With a smudge brush or a lining brush, smudge the outside top line of eyeliner so it's not a straight line but a blurred one. Try to blend it in with that darkest color that is on your lid.

STEP 8: Curl your dry lashes with an eyelash curler before applying the mascara.

STEP 9: Mascara the hell out of your upper and lower lashes. Too much is never enough. Less is not more!

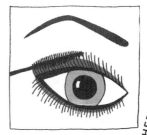

CHERRY BOMB

STEP 10: Makeup artists never do this, but I do and it works great: After the mascara has dried, I curl my lashes again with the eyelash curler. Don't forget to wash your curler between uses.

STEP 11: With eyes this dramatic, chances are you'll need to fill in your eyebrows a bit to balance it out.

Remember! You might have to go over each color a few times to achieve the desired shade and to be blended to perfection. Colors look different on different skin tones, so expect to spend a little bit of time tweaking. Go slowly. Take your time. This isn't an easy makeup trick to pull off.

𝔉AKE IT!

If you want a more dramatic look, fake eyelashes are the way to go. If you have the money, go for lash extensions. They can cost between $250 and $350, but they are incredibly natural looking and will have you looking fab-u-LASH for about a month. If that's not in the budget, then get M.A.C.'s Lash 1. It's a more natural fake lash than some of the others. When you buy them at the M.A.C. store, ask one of the on-site makeup artists to apply them for you, and pay attention so you can learn how to apply them yourself. (The service is free!)

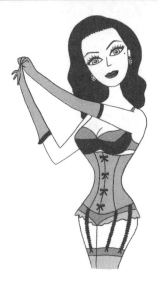

STRIPTEASE

𝕭𝖞 𝖇𝖚𝖗𝖑𝖊𝖘𝖖𝖚𝖊 𝖘𝖙𝖆𝖗 𝕯𝖎𝖙𝖆 𝖁𝖔𝖓 𝕿𝖊𝖊𝖘𝖊

"Hello, fellow sex bombs! As you may know, I'm notoriously adept at taking off my clothes in a skillful manner onstage. But what you may not know is that I love using some of my skills in the bedroom from time to time for my most deserving lovers! So, what you have here are some suggestions for successfully performing an intimate seductive striptease. They are merely suggestions, not rules, so use these little pearls of wisdom as you wish. But don't forget to try out some moves of your own, and above all, let your own character and charisma shine through.

ꙅUITING UP

The first thing you'll need is the perfect lingerie. If you're planning on getting down and dirty, forget the nipple tassels. They were invented for burlesque in the 1930s because the cops were lurking about, and showing your naughty bits was illegal. But in this case, there are no limits, so keep your boobies glue-free and you will thank me later!

The ideal lingerie for a striptease consists of a bra, a garter belt, stockings, and panties. The idea is to have lots of layers that can effortlessly be removed slowly in order to work your victim into a tantalizing tizzy. Choose lingerie that fits you well and makes *you* feel sexy. Don't think too much about what your target would prefer; a successful strip is about exuding confidence and sensuality, so focus on the kind of clothing that makes you feel that way.

Now, personally, I'm a girl who knows the power of black lace and black sheer seamed stockings. This seems to work every time! (Go to www.dita.net for shopping links to some of my favorite lingerie designers.) Some of my favorites are Agent Provocateur, Victoria's Secret, www.secretsinlace.com, Mr. Pearl, Chantal Thomass, Dark Garden Corsetry and Trashy Lingerie, and my vintage-inspired lingerie by Wonderbra. Here is what to look for when shopping:

THE CLOTHES: Before we get to the lingerie, let's talk about what to wear *over* your undergarments. A sexy suit or skirt-and-blouse combination is ideal. Look for pieces that cover your lingerie and don't reveal too much at first. I love a suit! Things that unbutton down the front are perfect. Finding a skirt that wraps around to close is a dream come true! Whatever you choose, you need to slip out of it effortlessly and elegantly. No back zippers that are too high for you to reach and nothing that comes off over your head. You don't want to mess up your hair or get stuck!

THE BRA: I like a bra with side shoulder straps and that pushes my breasts up but is not too heavily padded.

THE GARTER BELT: In my day-to-day life, I prefer a wide and substantial garter belt to keep my stockings in place. But in the case of a private striptease with someone *ahem* special, I go for something more svelte. You might find that the striptease ends abruptly at about the time the panties come off (go figure!), so the garter belt choice is vital! It is important to choose a garter belt with metal clips, not plastic. And don't even think about buying one with those silly metal alligator teeth clips to hold the stockings up. Buy the real deal and practice hooking and unhooking those clips until it becomes second nature.

THE STOCKINGS: First, note that stockings are not the same as "panty hose." Stockings do not come up to the waist. They stop midthigh and attach to a garter belt. That said, in this day and age, great stockings aren't so easy to come by. Do not choose thigh-high, rubberized stockings. Your garter belt clips will not hook to them properly, and they aren't as sexy as the real deal. Thigh-highs also pinch into your thighs—not pretty. You really have two options here, and both have their advantages. Let me explain . . .

The first option is fully fashioned nylon seamed stockings. These look the best and feel the sexiest, and you will appear to be a dame who knows her stuff. There is nothing quite like the rasp of true nylon against the skin. (Silk stockings are nearly impossible to find and tend to get baggy, so don't waste time tracking them down for this.) And the details of vintage-styled stockings are beautiful and sexy, and if your "audience" happens to be a foot or stockings enthusiast, I promise you that this choice will make you unforgettable! You can get the Dita Von Teese brand at www.secretsinlace.com.

The second option is nylon stockings with a touch of Lycra. This is a slightly more user-friendly method. They won't get wrinkles, they probably won't run as easily, and you can do tricks with these, like pulling them off in clever ways or flinging them about the room. But you will be missing that soft, delicate, wispy feel that you get with a true nylon stocking. But why not try both?

The best bit of stocking advice? Buy *two* pairs of each style/color. If you run one, the pair isn't history; you still have a spare! My best suggestion is to practice with both kinds of stockings and see which one you have the most fun with. Oh, and if you plan on having sex, tuck a condom into your stocking top. It gets the point across in a sexy way. And don't forget, safe sex is sexy!

THE PANTIES: Are you a thong girl or a briefs girl? Personally, I go for the bikini brief because I want each and every reveal to have a major impact, so if your rear end is covered completely and you peel the panty off, you are going to get a great reaction at the sudden sight of

CHERRY BOMB

your naked bum! If you want to get really fancy, wear a thong under your panty, and you have yet another fabulous layer to reveal. Now, take these next words of wisdom and use them for the rest of your life: Wear your panties OVER your garter belt. Always! It's absolutely silly to wear them any other way, you never know when you will want quick access, and furthermore, I have yet to meet a man who doesn't enjoy the sight of a woman in nothing but a garter and stockings! When shopping for panties, you might even get lucky and find something with side ties or hooks. Not a bad idea, but I still prefer the "bend over ever so slightly and slide them down" trick.

THE SHOES: Choose shoes that are as high as you can handle without falling over. Go for a shoe that slips off easily rather than a shoe with straps or buckles. Or, if the shoes are supersexy but too hard to walk in, try crawling. It's fun and naughty!

THE GLOVES: Any length gloves will do, but opera length, which come up to the upper arm, are classic. The gloves should come off first in your striptease. In burlesque, a dancer taking off her glove is really about the promise of what's to come.

CHECKLIST BEFORE GOING FOR IT: *Wax or shave your bikini area and legs. Get a manicure and pedicure. Make sure your hair and makeup are done up and sexy. (I like soft curls or waves best.) And make sure every inch of your body is primed, beautiful, and deliciously scented.*

SETTING THE TONE

THE MIND-SET: The first thing to do is to get yourself in the right mood. Do what it takes to put yourself in a sexy state of mind, because as we all know, you need to genuinely feel sexy in yourself before anyone else can see you as truly sexy. If you don't believe in yourself, why should others? If a cocktail makes you feel more at ease, have one or two. Not three or four. A bit of *ivresse*, which is a fabulous French word for that very light feeling of happiness that sweeps over you when drinking champagne, is acceptable. But being a sloppy, drunken mess is not.

THE LIGHTING: I cannot express the importance of proper lighting enough! I have dimmer switches in every room of my house, and I'm not exaggerating. Every single room! If you can't dim the lights, you can use candlelight or softly drape the lights with a scarf. I would choose a deep pink or lavender for the most flattering tones. Naked ladies look prettiest bathed in rose pink light! Red can be a little too harsh.

THE MUSIC: Choose music that *you* personally love. I can't tell you what music is going to put you in the mood; that is up to you. If you want some musical suggestions, see the sidebar below. But, ultimately, you should choose music from any era that suits your personality. Are you a slow seductress or a fiery bombshell? Do you want to do it wild, fierce, and fast? Or are you more the slow, seductive, and sensual type? If rap music puts you in the mood, choose a good rap song. You probably only need one long song, but I suggest having a second one ready just in case you're not quite there yet.

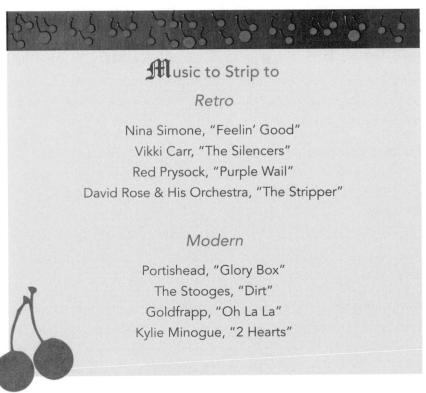

𝔐usic to Strip to

Retro

Nina Simone, "Feelin' Good"
Vikki Carr, "The Silencers"
Red Prysock, "Purple Wail"
David Rose & His Orchestra, "The Stripper"

Modern

Portishead, "Glory Box"
The Stooges, "Dirt"
Goldfrapp, "Oh La La"
Kylie Minogue, "2 Hearts"

THE VICTIM: Once you're looking gorgeous in your outfit, the music is ready, and the lights are dim, you want to make your victim comfortable in a cozy chair or sofa. If he likes a drink, provide his favorite. This is a special occasion, after all! If he is a handsy fellow (or a handsy *lady* if that is your desire), consider tying his hands with a silk tie or those stockings you ripped during your rehearsal. We don't want him or her spoiling all the fun by throwing you over his or her shoulder and taking you to the bedroom just yet, do we? (Or do we?) The choice is yours. Hazard of the profession, indeed!

THE CHAIR: Place a chair for yourself directly across from him about four or five feet away. Choose a chair that feels stable to you—you get extra points for a pretty chair, like a parlor chair or upholstered chair that complements your lingerie!

⚔AKING IT OFF

I can't necessarily give you a play-by-play on how to do a striptease, because anything really does go and there are no hard rules. Don't overthink it; feel it and just go with it. Make your own rules. That said I will get you started by giving you some pointers and some of my personal tried-and-true tricks and tips. Consider these merely to be suggestions. Okay, here we go:

PRACTICE AND PLAN: Practice does make perfect, so take what I say here and spend some time in front of a mirror to see what works best for you and really see how your body looks in these moves. Adjust it as needed. Plant it out. You don't want to look choreographed, but plotting it out in your head (and in front of the mirror) before you do it will really help. Think ahead of time about what you want to take off first and where you want to end up.

FIRST THINGS FIRST: The gloves should come off first (it's easier to unhook your bra later with your bare hands than with gloved hands). You can take the gloves off with your teeth and toss them his way. After the gloves are off, anything goes. You can take your suit jacket off first, or you can take off the skirt or dress. Do what feels natural to you. Tease with a flash of garter before taking the skirt or dress off, though.

HAT TRICKS: If you want to wear a hat, a good move would be to hold the hat in front of your boobs with one hand and then, with the other hand, slip your bra off behind it. Toss the bra aside and put both hands on your hat, hiding your bare breasts. Then turn around to show your naked back and turn back around to take the hat away from your breasts for your reveal. Go slowly and make him wait for it.

SMOOTH MOVES: Your movements as you strip away each article of clothing should be slow, graceful, and deliberate, but not forced. And you should think about exaggerating your curves in every move. For example, if you have one knee bent, pull your tummy in, sit up straight so your chest is out, and stick your butt out. It's all about those curves, so work them! Shaking boobs or booty is okay. Try to keep it sexy but not raunchy or vulgar.

TOUCH YOURSELF: Sometimes the smallest gesture, say a touch to your own neck or your hair, can really turn him on. Make eye contact with him while you do this. When all else fails, touch yourself. Give yourself a little caress. Try tracing your silhouette: Outline your breasts with your hand and move down to your waist and hips. Trace your body and follow your lines in pretty, soft moves—don't go for raunchy boob-grabbing here. Save that for later!

TALK TO YOURSELF: I have an inner monologue going when I do my striptease. It's just a simple, "Okay, now I'm taking my bra off. Here comes the bra. Now I'm revealing my breasts. Oooh. What do you think?" silently to myself. It helps me to pace out what I'm doing and to focus on the stripping and to let my inner thoughts come through my movements.

TALK DIRTY TO HIM: It's also fun to tease him with your words. You can say things such as, "Are you ready for a little treat?" "Do you see something you like?" "Should I take this off or leave it on?" "Do you want to see more?" "I bet you'd like to touch me, but you have to earn the right." "Wait like a good boy."

CHERRY BOMB

LETTING YOUR HAIR DOWN: Taking your hair down can be just as sexy as taking your clothes off. First, make sure you perfume your hair. Spray a little on your hairbrush and brush it through your locks. Spray some on the nape of your neck too. Try putting your hair in a little chignon with one simple hair clip or one large hairpin and let it down at just the right moment. Play with your hair, toss it around, and shake it out. Men love gorgeous hair.

DISCARDING THE CLOTHES: It's fun to toss a bra or a glove at your man, but it'll get boring if you toss every piece of clothing you take off. Try putting your arm out to your side and dropping the item on the floor, or bend over and place it on a chair. Mix it up and be creative. Treat whatever piece of clothing you remove as something special. But I am all for underwear flinging—especially if it lands on the chandelier or on a lamp.

PANTY REMOVAL: Careful underwear removal is important. Start in a standing position with your back to him. Keep grounded and steady. Hook your thumbs into each side of your panties, bend over to give him a lovely view of your butt, and pull the panties down.

When the panties hit the floor, stand up very carefully and slowly and step out of them. Then I like to bend over to pick them up off the floor, and maybe hand them to him.

LAST BUT NOT LEAST: The heels should come off last or not at all, depending on how you and your man like it. If you do take off your heels, the best way to do that without falling over is to sit in your chair (sit up straight—good posture makes your chest and butt stick out, and accentuating the curves is what we're going for), cross your legs, and let the shoe dangle on your foot before it falls to the floor. If it's comfortable for you, extend your other leg and maybe gently flick the shoe off your foot. (Don't forget to point your toes when doing this. *Always* point your toes—it's prettier that way.)

HAPPY ENDINGS: You can end your striptease completely naked or in any combination of clothing items you want. I find it's sexy to end the tease in nothing but heels and a garter belt. After that, well, you know what to do next . . . !

And, as we say in burlesque, break a leg!

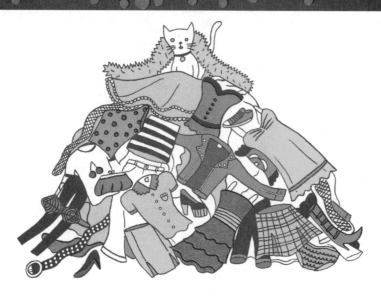

STYLE

Chances are you're like me and you flip through the pages of fashion magazines, celebrity weeklies, and women's magazines to check out what cool new looks your favorite celebrities are wearing. Staying on top of the latest trends and seeing what your favorite designers have in store for the new season is a big part of being a rocking style maven.

But don't fall into the trap of trying to look like these stars and re-duplicating those carefully styled outfits in *Vogue*. Why? You'll look like everyone else, and that is not what style is all about. Style is about expressing yourself as an individual. It's about finding what's unique in you and bringing it out. Style is about showing how you are different from everyone else.

The goal is to create your own look. The best thing to do if you're looking for a more rockin' new look is to mess around with some style staples from past eras. A great way to be fashion forward is to look back, as everything old becomes new again at some point.

Gwen Stefani and Amy Winehouse are great examples of women who mix the past with the present to create unique looks all their own.

CHERRY BOMB

Gwen takes risks by playing around with patterns (her faves being houndstooth, leopard, and stripes), pairing punky plaid pants with a classic, sleek trench, or wearing a '50s black leather jacket and leather studded belt with a '60s miniskirt—and always with her Old Hollywood platinum locks and red lips. Amy takes a '50s beehive and pairs it with '60s heavy black eyeliner and a modern pair of skinny jeans with some indie rock sneakers and an '80s preppy Polo shirt. Talk about crossing genres. But it works!

Check out the popular style essentials from past eras below. Select a few of your favorite items, then raid your closet and see how they go together.

1940S

PENCIL SKIRTS

FINGERWAVES OR PIN CURLS IN THE HAIR

STOCKINGS

LADYLIKE BLOUSES

PUMPS

1950S

FULL SKIRTS

TIGHT CASHMERE SWEATERS

BEEHIVE HAIR OR PONYTAILS

PEDAL PUSHERS

BLACK LEATHER JACKETS

1960S

THE MOD LOOK: minidresses, go-go boots, black liquid eyeliner, and Pucci

MINISKIRTS

BABY-DOLL DRESSES

A-LINE DRESSES

THE HIPPY LOOK: tie-dye, hip-hugger bell-bottoms, peasant blouses, and vests

1970S

FLARED JEANS

LEATHER AND SUEDE

DISCO: spandex, polyester, hot pants, lamé, and shiny Lycra

GLAM ROCK: androgynous looks, boas, glitter, silver, and heavy makeup

PLATFORM SHOES

PUNK ROCK: plaid, studded belts, torn clothes, vinyl, bondage-wear, and Mohawks

1980S

LEGGINGS

ASYMMETRICAL HAIR, TOPS, AND DRESSES

STRIPES AND NEON

THE PREPPY LOOK

STILETTOS

SKINNY JEANS

GOTH: all black, corsets, fishnets, and Victorian and Elizabethan styles

12 FASHION TIPS
BY ROCK STYLIST CYNTHIA FREUND
(TOMMY LEE, NIKKI SIXX, DAVE NAVARRO)

1 LOVE THYSELF: Know what works for your body and buy pieces that fit and work for your own unique size and shape. Good undergarments are key too. Nothing kills a good look like an unsightly bulge in the wrong place.

2 DO RESEARCH: I collect tear sheets (pages torn from magazines) of outfits that I like and file them. When I get stumped in the morning while getting dressed, I pull them out to give me ideas of what to wear that day.

3 BE YOURSELF: Tommy Lee has a saying: "Be yourself . . . everyone else is already taken." I like that. I always say, "You have to wear your

CHERRY BOMB

179

clothes. Your clothes can't wear you." Keep both in mind. And don't buy the entire outfit off a mannequin, or dress head-to-toe in one designer (unless you are sponsored by that brand!). You need to mix it up with your individuality.

4 **BREAK THE RULES:** Real rock stars break all the fashion rules. Stripes and plaids, leather and lace, gold and silver. Mix it all up. And forget about that "no white after Labor Day" rule. My rock stars wear white all year round.

5 **GRRRRR. MIX, DON'T MATCH:** Remember the line Garanimals that made you match up the animals to create an outfit that goes together? It was extremely popular in the '70s. Well, those days are gone (though Garanimals are apparently still around . . . who knew, right?). Avoid being too matchy-matchy. No one matches their belt with their shoes anymore. Your toe polish doesn't need to match your shoe color. And purses should complement your outfit but not necessarily match it exactly.

6 **HIT THE MALL:** For inexpensive rocker chick clothing, I like to go to mall shops like Forever 21, Hot Topic, and Wet Seal for trendy designer knockoffs. To add my own individuality, I finish up the look with items I get at swap meets. One person's trash can be another person's treasure. And who knew Grandma's jewels, Dad's socks, and some stranger's twelve-year-old-sister's hat would look so cute together, but sometimes they do. Mix it up. With all the money you'll save, you can treat yourself to an expensive designer handbag.

 Fun Fact: *The red minidress that Gwen Stefani wore on the cover of No Doubt's CD* Tragic Kingdom *was purchased at mall store Contempo Casuals for a mere $14. So cheap and chic, even for 1995!*

7 SHOP VINTAGE: Vintage shopping is best in the ritzier areas of bigger cities. That's where all the "fancy pants" ladies dump their designer pieces or custom-made outfits on a regular basis. Celebs don't like wearing the same outfit twice, especially if they get photographed a lot, so they end up unloading a lot of stuff at vintage or consignment shops.

> " I had a very limited budget to work with when I started out in the band, so I made some of my clothes, and we would go to crazy places to shop. I lived on the Bowery, in New York, and there were lots of what we called 'the bum stores,' where the vagrants would sell all manner of junk that they had just picked up, at really cheap prices. I bought some interesting T-shirts there, and some really cool heavy framed square sunglasses that were like something out of a cartoon."
>
> ~DEBBIE HARRY OF BLONDIE *(TIMES ONLINE U.K.)*

8 IT'S OK TO SPLURGE: A good deal is really relative to your budget. If you really love something, then any amount is justifiable because the happiness that the item can bring you is priceless.

9 DECONSTRUCT: My rock stars like designer duds, but they LOVE designer duds when I fuck them up for them. I rip and fray all the seams on Gucci pants for Nikki Sixx. I cut the sleeves off Dolce & Gabbana shirts for Dave Navarro. And I completely deconstruct Hugo Boss suits for Tommy Lee. Mixing designer clothes with each of their individual street styles is key to my rock star styling. And, yes, this works for women's wear too, and you can create these looks with lower-end brands as well.

10 EDIT YOUR ACCESSORIES: Don't overdo it. If you're wearing a lot of necklaces, you might not want to wear bracelets or rings or a big belt as well. Learn to edit yourself.

11 TOOLS OF THE TRADE: The top two supplies that can save you in a fashion emergency are top stick (aka double-stick tape) and black safety pins. I use top stick to tape collars down or to secure fabric to skin so you don't have any peek-a-boo moments on the red carpet that end up on "Page Six." I use black safety pins (if you can't find them, you can spray-paint regular pins) when tape isn't strong enough. I sometimes pin the clothing in a way that makes a fashion statement. Combining fashion with function is very punk rock.

⓬ CLEAN HOUSE: I edit my closet every six months and have a yard sale where I sell each item for $5. Five-dollar bills add up! I usually get rid of superboring pieces or supertrendy pieces. I keep the unique ones forever. Some items come back into style after a while, so hang on to the interesting pieces to start your own vintage collection.

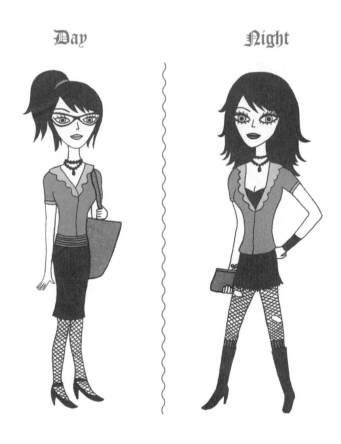

Day   Night

CYNTHIA'S TIPS ON ROCKING UP YOUR DAYTIME WORK OUTFIT FOR A NIGHT ON THE TOWN

If you wear casual clothes to work, like jeans and a T-shirt, you can simply put on some heels and add some fun accessories like a belt, a scarf, a hat, or cool jewelry and you're ready to rock.

If you are a real rock star, you can take some scissors to your T-shirt and make a halter or tube top out of it. Then, take the scrap fabric from the top and make it into a wrist or leg band.

If you wear fancy clothes to work, like a button-down shirt, skirt, and stockings, just unbutton a few more buttons or strip down to the sexy camisole you have underneath and cut or burn holes in your stockings. Then throw on a pair of knee socks over them and put on some boots.

If you wear your hair up during the day, take it down and wear it messy. If you wear it down, put it up in a sloppy bun.

Eyeliner is a must with all of the above outfits. It's the best way to "sexy up" any look and the quickest way to go from daytime look to evening.

HOW A PRO LIKE CYNTHIA HANDLES A FASHION EMERGENCY

I was at the Comedy Central Roast of Pamela Anderson with my client Tommy Lee. At the after-party, Tommy brought Pam over to me and said, "Baby, help! We got a fashion emergency!" I looked at Pam's dress, and the zipper in the back had completely ripped out. I assessed the situation and asked Tommy to find a pocketknife. He did in seconds flat. (I didn't even want to know how!) I took the knife and punctured holes down each side of the fabric where the zipper was. Then I gathered everyone's VIP lanyards, which were made of metal beads, and hooked them all together. I laced up Pam's dress with it and, voila! A corseted look for the lady of the evening.

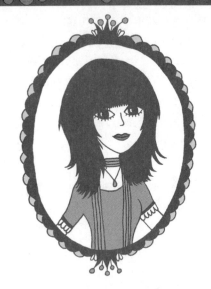

ANNA SUI

What Makes Anna Sui Rock?

urple and black. Velvet and ruffles. Japanese anime and dolly heads. Hippie chic and '70s glam rock. These are the things that Anna Sui's designs are made of. And of all the designers who rock stars love, Anna Sui is probably the designer who loves rock stars back the most.

The Chinese-American Sui (born in Birmingham, Michigan) has made a name for herself by infusing her love for all eras of rock and roll into her designs. Not surprisingly, Sui, a self-proclaimed rock chick who was a regular on the underground punk scene in New York in the '70s and whose favorite bands include the Rolling Stones, the White Stripes, and the Greenhorns, turns her runway shows into rock shows by blaring rock, punk, and glam songs as edgy models strut their stuff. She's even had rock stars, like the Smashing Pumpkins' guitarist James Iha, walk for her.

Her designs are flirty but tough, vintage-inspired but modern, and easy to wear to a concert, a movie date, or a walk through the park.

In 1998, she presented her Goth collection, which she said was inspired by her friendship with the Cure's Robert Smith, with models wearing makeup a la Goth queen Siouxsie Sioux and walking down the catwalk to the music of Bauhaus. "When I started designing, my intention was to dress rock stars and people who went to rock concerts . . . and that's what I still do. Music has always been a major influence on me. I've worked many rock themes into my work: punk, glam, Goth, folk, mod, grunge, and psychedelia," explains Sui.

In 2006, Mattel commemorated Sui's Bohemian hippie chick look with a limited edition Anna Sui Boho Barbie. She switched genres again for her spring 2007 collection, which she has described as a mix of eighteenth-century influences with a punk rock attitude, like "Glitter-Rock Marie Antoinette Swashbuckler." And spring 2008 saw her love of '70s glam mixed with Hollywood glamour of the '30s and '40s with a collection that cited as her muses famous music groupies Sable Starr and Cyrinda Foxe and Andy Warhol "stars" Jane Forth and Donna Jordan.

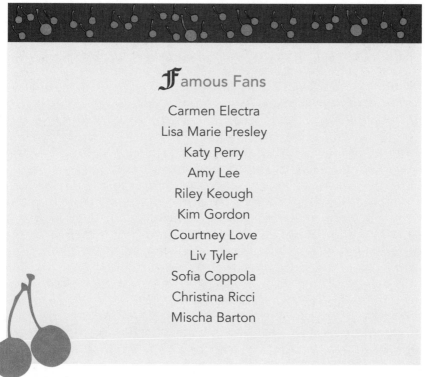

𝕱amous Fans

Carmen Electra
Lisa Marie Presley
Katy Perry
Amy Lee
Riley Keough
Kim Gordon
Courtney Love
Liv Tyler
Sofia Coppola
Christina Ricci
Mischa Barton

𝔉OUR QUESTIONS FOR ANNA SUI

How does music inspire your designs?

Usually when I'm designing, I like to listen to music that puts me in the mood. Sometimes I listen to the Cure or Bob Dylan, but lately I've been playing a lot of Joy Division, the Clash, and the Beatles. The Rolling Stones were always my favorite style icons; I always incorporate elements of their look into my personal wardrobe and into what I design for my collection (pinstriped pants, ruffled shirts, tall boots).

What advice do you have for a girl who is trying to develop her own personal style?

Make an effort, opt for a little glamour, experiment with new ideas, have some fun, and don't take yourself so seriously.

Who are your favorite rock chicks today?

The Donnas, Cat Power, and Karen O from Yeah Yeah Yeahs. They characterize the look of the contemporary version of a rock and roll girl; it's all about the attitude.

What are your favorite vintage stores around the world?

What Comes Around Goes Around and Cherry in New York; Resurrection in New York and Los Angeles; Portobello Road Flea Market (particularly on Friday mornings) in London; and Vali Folkart Antique in Budapest, Hungary.

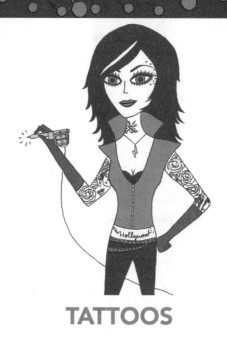

TATTOOS

By L.A. Ink star/tattoo artist Kat Von D.

7 THINGS TO THINK ABOUT BEFORE GETTING A TATTOO

1 TRAMP STAMPS: I think tramp stamps became popular mainly because people who were in the public eye, such as Britney Spears, Drew Barrymore, and Christina Aguilera, were getting them done. Plus I feel like tattoos, especially on women, should accentuate the body. And what more feminine place than the lower back? Whenever I see someone with a "tramp stamp," I automatically think of doing it "doggy style" (I'm pretty sure most guys do too). So when my mom asked me to give her her first tattoo, I was stoked but bummed out at the same time that she wanted it on her lower back. The last thing I want to do is picture my mom having sex, let alone doing it doggy style!

2 DON'T BE TRENDY: Getting a certain design or image tattooed on your body that is in or popular at the moment is not always the wisest choice when it comes to picking out your tattoo, because, just like any other fad, trends eventually go out of style. Because tattoos are permanent, this is not a good idea.

3 FOREIGN WORDS & SYMBOLS: Doing research before getting a tattoo is important. If you're getting lettering tattooed in a language that's foreign to you, make sure you're getting the word or phrase from a reliable source. The Internet makes it a lot easier to get accurate translations, but even then online translations can have mistakes. Clients oftentimes want to get words, say, in Japanese kanji or in Chinese, and my best advice is to take a little trip to Chinatown if you have one in your city (San Francisco, Los Angeles, and New York have them) and find a lettering expert who specializes in brushstroke calligraphy. Ask them to give you an accurate translation, but also make it unique and cool-looking so your tattoo won't just look like a font taken from the Internet.

4 LOVERS' NAMES: I have mixed feelings about this subject in particular because not only was my first tattoo the initial of the boyfriend I had at the time, but I've since added several more boyfriends' names to the collection, as well as my husband's name, initials, and a portrait of someone I'm no longer with. Yeah, it sucks to wake up every morning and have a constant reminder of a love that once was, but I don't regret those landmarks in time. Nowadays, with the advance of laser tattoo removal and tattoo artists' skills, it's a lot easier to either remove a tattoo or cover it with another one. Some see getting lovers' names tattooed on their bodies as a curse, but I for one say live and learn.

5 DO IT SOBER: Making decisions on important matters such as getting a tattoo should never be made while your judgment is impaired by any substances, such as alcohol. That's just a no-brainer. There's nothing worse than waking up with a hangover and a tattoo that you don't remember getting, let alone one that's spelled wrong.

6 BE ORIGINAL: Tattoos are known to be a form of self-expression. Being unique is always a good thing. Don't get me wrong, everyone has their influences, but I think most clients are far happier when they get something custom made just for them.

7 PAY UP: Some of the best advice when it comes to this subject is one of the oldest rules in the book: "You get what you pay for." Getting a tattoo shouldn't be like bargaining at a swap meet. This is something that you are going to wear on your body for the rest of your life. Good tattoos aren't cheap, and cheap tattoos aren't good. Period.

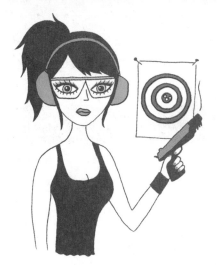

> *Girls have got balls. They're just a little higher up, that's all."*
> ~JOAN JETT

TOUGH CHICKS

10 STEPS TO BECOMING A TOUGHER CHICK

1 Take a self-defense class and learn how to flip a man twice your size over your shoulder.

2 Call that bitch out on her evil ways to her face.

3 Learn how to change your own flat tire.

4 Take charge of the grill at the next BBQ instead of having your boyfriend, father, or brother handle the "manly duty" of cooking meat.

5 Passionately throw him up against the wall for once.

6 Say "Are you talking to me?" at least once in your life, in a bar, to someone much larger than you.

7 Dress up and act like anyone on the list of Famous Tough Chicks on the next page for your next costume party . . . or just for a fun night in with your man!

8 Hit the shooting range and learn how to fire a gun. Just don't go all Thelma and Louise on us.

CHERRY BOMB

9 Take up kickboxing.

10 Take a page out of Carrie Underwood's book (i.e., her pro-girl anthem "Before He Cheats") and learn to shoot whiskey and how to shoot a combo.

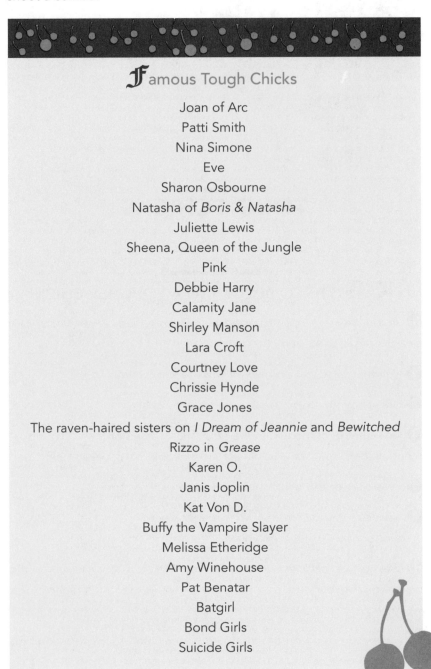

Famous Tough Chicks

Joan of Arc
Patti Smith
Nina Simone
Eve
Sharon Osbourne
Natasha of *Boris & Natasha*
Juliette Lewis
Sheena, Queen of the Jungle
Pink
Debbie Harry
Calamity Jane
Shirley Manson
Lara Croft
Courtney Love
Chrissie Hynde
Grace Jones
The raven-haired sisters on *I Dream of Jeannie* and *Bewitched*
Rizzo in *Grease*
Karen O.
Janis Joplin
Kat Von D.
Buffy the Vampire Slayer
Melissa Etheridge
Amy Winehouse
Pat Benatar
Batgirl
Bond Girls
Suicide Girls

THE ULTIMATE TOUGH CHICK SOUNTRACK

1. The Runaways, "Cherry Bomb"

2. Joan Jett & the Blackhearts, "Bad Reputation"

3. Pat Benatar, "Hit Me with Your Best Shot"

4. Peaches, "Boys Wanna Be Her"

5. Veruca Salt, "Volcano Girls"

6. Garbage, "Supervixen"

7. Hole, "Violet"

8. Donna Summer, "Bad Girls"

9. Blondie, "Call Me"

10. Heart, "Barracuda"

CHERRY BOMB

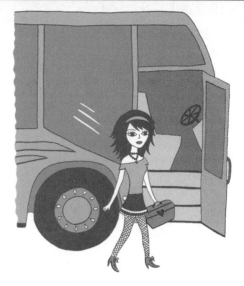

TOUR BUS ETIQUETTE

A TOUR BUS HAIKU

Tour bus can be fun,
If you follow certain rules,
Can go one, not two!

our buses are fun. They're basically a bar, a dance club, and a lounge on wheels. What isn't fun about that? I'll tell you what's not fun—having the singer, tour manager, or bitchy band wife snap at you for doing something wrong. Follow these rules of the road and you won't get kicked to the curb.

❶ Just like *Fight Club* and partying in Las Vegas, what happens on the bus stays on the bus.

❷ Bathrooms on most buses can only take number one. Some buses have a grinder for number two. Make sure you ask first what your bathroom is equipped for before dropping trou. Most likely, it won't have a grinder for number two. So, if nature's calling and you really can't hold it, you need to ask the person you're with to ask the driver to pull over at the next truck stop. If you just have to go number one,

CARRIE BORZILLO-VRENNA

take note: The toilet paper goes in the trash bag, not down the bowl. And remember, being proactive can save your ass (literally), so don't eat tummy-stirring food before you go on the bus; that way you can avoid having to pull over.

3 A sippy cup is your friend. Being drunk on a bus with an open cup is a recipe for disaster—if you spill on someone's bunk or in the lounge that everyone shares, there will be hell to pay.

4 Knock before entering the back lounge. You don't want to walk in on someone having sex.

5 Ask someone else to get you a drink from the refrigerator. Opening the refrigerator door while the bus is moving and having the contents come flying out at you is embarrassing. Trust me. And if you're not experienced at this, it WILL happen to you.

6 Don't get the driver high.

7 If your bus stops in the middle of the night and you hear dogs barking, flush (or ingest) any illegal substances you may have.

8 The singer always gets first choice of what to watch or listen to on the bus. Know your band hierarchy—singer ranks first, songwriting guitarist second, bassist third, drummer fourth, band wives next, and band girlfriends last. Guests don't get to dictate what goes on the tube.

9 Don't accidentally drink the ashtray. Most people on the bus use a water bottle as an ashtray, so before you grab a bottle of H_2O and start chugging, take a look and make sure it's not where the smokers are ashing their butts. (I learned that the hard way. See the sidebar on the next page.)

10 Ask before you eat the band's food. The band hates when a guest eats the food they were saving for a late-night snack.

11 If the band members aren't smoking but you *must* smoke a cigarette, go up front into the jump seat next to the driver and open the passenger window to have a cig.

⑫ Don't sit in the front lounge and talk loudly on your cell phone. The band doesn't want to hear your chitchat, especially after playing a long show. Only use your phone if it's an emergency, and even then, be sure to be quiet and quick.

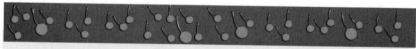

𝔐y True Story:
Making an Ash out of Myself!

A few years ago, I was whooping it up one night in the back lounge of the tour bus with my husband and a few band members. It was one of those bus rides between shows that isn't long enough to sleep in our cozy little bunks but isn't short enough to NOT start drinking heavily. So, the drinking began—made even easier, faster, and much more dangerous by the fact that I was drinking absinthe out of the sippy cup I got at the Rock & Roll Hall of Fame in Cleveland the day before. The sippy cup was helping the absinthe go down, and my hubby couldn't keep up with my refill requests. We were singing along to someone's iPod, and I was oblivious to all around me and feeling dehydrated. I entered the back lounge and took a huge swig out of what I thought was my water bottle. Before I could taste what was happening, I saw it on everyone's faces and heard my husband yell, "Babe . . . nooooo!" in that *Matrix* slo-mo kind of way. But it was too late. I had taken a swig not from my water bottle but from the bottle that everyone was using as their ashtray. To this day, I blame it on the sippy cup!

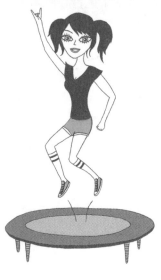

TRAMPING

No, tramping does not mean acting like a whore. Tramping is what I dubbed my rock chick workout.

I hate the gym. I hate gym clothes. I hate sneakers. I hate buff, muscular, jarhead men asking to spot me or saying "Looking good." So I came up with a fun way to work out at home. Simply put, "tramping" means to rock out on your mini trampoline to your favorite tunes. And it also happens to be a fun cardio workout (just ask Dita Von Teese, who tramps to keep in shape as well, or my friend Mollie Johnson, who's a yoga instructor).

No matter how small your apartment is, I know you have room for a miniature trampoline, which has a mere 38-inch radius and stands only nine inches high. You can fit it under a bed, in a closet, or lean it up behind the couch. And I also know you have the budget for one. Most mini tramps cost about $50, and you can buy them online.

Here's how to rock it:

SET UP

■ Close your blinds and windows. (Unless you're an exhibitionist!)

■ Take off your shoes. Feel free to wear socks or go barefoot.

CHERRY BOMB

195

■ Put on your favorite rock chick album. I often use greatest hits collections by Pat Benatar, Joan Jett, or Blondie. Turn it up loud.

WARM UP

■ With your feet hip-width apart and your arms bent as they would be if you were jogging, slowly jog in place for one song.

■ Once you're used to the spring-action underneath you, pick up the speed so that you are now running in place instead of jogging. Gradually lift your knees higher as you pick up speed. Keep this up for a few songs.

ROCK OUT

■ Pump your fist in the air above your head as if you're at the coliseum rocking out to a metal band. Pump ten times with your right arm and then ten times with your left. (Good for those "bingo wings"—you know, the arm flab that flaps back and forth when old ladies clap at bingo.)

■ With your arms bent at your sides, extend one fist straight out in front of you. For inspiration, think of hitting your evil ex-boyfriend or your boss or the chick who called you chunky. Repeat on each side for one song.

■ Put your arms above your head with your palms touching each other and your elbows slightly bent, a la Christina Aguilera in the "Genie in a Bottle" video. With your feet together on the tramp, twist your body right to left, sticking your hip out to the right, then the left, back and forth. Do this for one song.

■ If you want to get your triceps going, add some Pete Townshend (of the Who) windmills in the mix as you are jogging.

CHILL OUT

■ Bring it back down to a slow jog for one final song.

"Mistakes are part of the dues one pays for a full life."

~SOPHIA LOREN

"A man who has committed a mistake and doesn't correct it is committing another mistake."

~CONFUCIUS

"Oops! . . . I Did It Again."

~BRITNEY SPEARS

UH-OHS

Everybody makes mistakes. But a rock chick knows not only how to recover but also how to make the mishap work in her favor. Here are a few helpful examples:

You call your lover John, and his name is Steve . . . and you're in bed. Don't let it put a damper on the fun. When he says, "Uh, my name is Steve," reply in your best sex-kitten voice, "Not tonight, dear. You're Johnny Depp." He'll be less likely to get mad at you if he thinks you're just engaging in a little harmless fantasizing.

You're talking smack about a bitchy broad and she hears you and asks, "Are you talking about me?" Of course, your first instinct is to just lie and say, "No." But if she really heard you, she'll stay the course and say, "But I heard my name. You said Kim!" You should then laugh and say, "Oh. Another Kim." Then go back to your conversation and keep talking about her as if nothing happened and as if you're really talking about a different person who just happens to have the same name.

You fall into the pool at a party. No worries. Take off all your clothes and start swimming as if you meant to do it. Hopefully, others will join in and then you'll be the life of the party instead of the fool who fell in.

You farted in bed. Don't pull a Carrie Bradshaw and scurry away as if nothing happened. Get it out in the open and just laugh about it with your partner. Or blame it on him!

You are way overdressed for a party. I mean waaaayyyy overdressed. You show up in a fluffy Betsey Johnson ruffle dress and everyone else is casual in jeans and T-shirts. Tell your fellow partiers that it's your birthday. If this crowd knows you too well for that cover-up, then tell them you went to a fabulous fancy event earlier and didn't have time to change.

You are superlate for a meeting. Don't rush in all flustered and apologizing. Walk in calm, cool, and collected and act surprised when you see the room is already full. Say, "Wow. We're all early." Pretend that you truly believe the meeting begins at 1:30 (even though it started at 1:00), and that you honestly think you are ten minutes early.

You get wasted at a work party or family gathering. And, yes, your coworkers/family members will be talking about it for years to come. Use the excuse celebrities abuse and say that you accidentally mixed prescription meds with alcohol. Just say you were taking an antibiotic for a dental issue and that you knew not to have that glass of champagne (or two or three), but you were having so much fun with your coworkers/family that you just lost your senses. Oopsie!

You royally fuck up with a boyfriend, a friend, a coworker, or a relative in a major way. It involves belligerent behavior in a public place and words that cut someone to the core. Write a formal apology letter. In your missive, give them the one-two-three punch. First, apologize for your inappropriate behavior, then admit one of three things—that you have an alcohol or drug problem that caused the outburst, that you were having an insecure moment and it's something you are working on, or (sorry feminists!) that you are hormonal because you are either PMSing or you might be pregnant. Then end with this: "It will never happen again. I hope you understand that that was not who I am, but just me at my worst on one bad night. I hope you will give me a second chance. But, if not, I understand." Most people will give a second chance—so don't F-up this royally again!

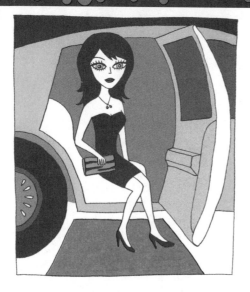

UNDIES

What you wear under your rocking outfits is just as important as the outfit itself. Proper undergarments can make or break an outfit—or a date, for that matter. Whether you're after hiding an unsightly belly bulge or you're looking for the perfect sexy lingerie to seduce your man in, this quickie on undies will give you the lowdown on delicates.

HOW TO EXIT WITHOUT DISPLAYING YOUR UNDIES (OR LACK OF)

Take note, Britney Spears, Lindsay Lohan, and Paris Hilton. To exit a vehicle the classy way, scoot to the edge of the car seat so you are lined up parallel to the door. Keep your knees together. When the door opens, put your outer leg out first, keeping your knees closed, and put your other leg out next. Stand, and look confident.

CHERRY BOMB

ESSENTIAL ITEMS	
FREDERICK'S OF HOLLYWOOD	Bombshell corsets, marabou slippers, and sexy Santa outfits for the holidays
VICTORIA'S SECRET	This is where you stock up on all of your basics—from push-up bras to wireless bras to strapless bras to basic briefs, everyday bikinis, boy shorts, and hip-huggers. (Skip the thongs. They are sooooo 1990s!)
SPANX	All of their body shapers are miracle workers, but the seamless shaping bodysuit, seamless midthigh shaper, and control-top fishnets should top your list.
TRASHY LINGERIE	Lingerie costumes such as a sexy nurse, dirty French maid, naughty policewoman, pinup girl, burlesque star, and many more
AGENT PROVOCATEUR	Sheer black (with a touch of pink) demi-bra and panties with garter belt set
MR. PEARL	This Paris-based designer (Mark Pullin) makes custom-made couture corsets that have been known to cinch down a select few from a 24-inch waist to 20 inches for a price that can be in the neighborhood of $50,000.

HOW TO MAKE YOUR B-CUPS LOOK LIKE D-CUPS

Chicken cutlets are the answer. The best are by NuBra, and you can get them online or at any major department store. They are called chicken cutlets because in their nude-colored, oblong, and rubbery form, they look like pieces of raw chicken breasts. They stick onto your breasts and

PURPOSE	FAMOUS FANS	THE DAMAGE
This is good for when you want to feel saucy all day long and *really* turn up the heat in the bedroom. If you're in the L.A. area, their flagship store on Hollywood Blvd. has a cool display of celebrity-designed corsets that have been donated over the years for their annual Lingerie Art Auction for charity. You can see corsets designed by Sharon Stone, Jessica Alba, Julianne Moore, and Dita Von Teese.	The previously mentioned celebs, plus Amanda Bynes and Alyssa Milano	$
This is where you purchase your everyday underwear collection.	The Angels, past and present—Heidi Klum, Gisele Bundchen, Karolina Kurkova, Adriana Lima	$
For slimming and body-shaping purposes. They smooth out your lovely lady lumps, flatten the tummy, suck in the back fat, and lift your behind.	Queen Latifah, Jennifer Lopez, Renee Zellweger, Gwyneth Paltrow, Hilary Duff, Oprah Winfrey, Dita Von Teese	$$
It's not just for Halloween but also for role-playing in the bedroom or going out to a fetish club.	Christina Aguilera, Pamela Anderson, Kirsten Dunst, Carmen Electra, Kate Hudson, Juliette Lewis	$$$
This is for special occasions—anniversaries, your first weekend away together, and your wedding night.	Vivienne Westwood and Malcolm McLaren (parents of cofounder Joseph Corre), Kylie Minogue, Christina Aguilera, Carmen Electra, Kate Moss, Maggie Gyllenhaal, Lily Allen, Jennifer Lopez, Fergie	$$$$
For photo shoots, music videos, movies, and ultra-high-fashion special occasions	Dita Von Teese, Kylie Minogue, Jerry Hall, Victoria Beckham	$$$$$

have a hook in the middle to achieve added cleavage. But they're not just for strapless and backless tops or dresses! When you want to look va-va-va-voom, wear the cutlets in addition to your corset, bustier, or push-up padded underwire bra, and it will make your B cups look like Ds. You'll have people wondering, "Did she get a boob job?!"

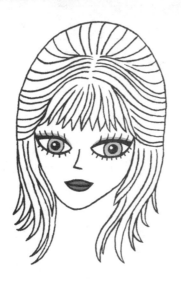
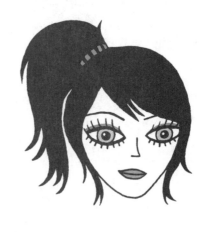

UP 'DOS

Too many great manes have been maimed by a hairdresser who still thinks an up 'do means that French twist you wore to your prom or involves ringlets of any kind. Save those for fancy-schmancy weddings. Here are two sexy and somewhat easy up 'dos for rockin' chicks to try instead, courtesy of Hollywood Hair Guy Dean Banowetz, who has worked his magic on the set of *American Idol* and is a hair expert/commentator for E!'s *Live from the Red Carpet*.

UP 'DO #1:
THE BRIGITTE BARDOT HALF-UP/HALF-DOWN

STEP 1: You want to begin by washing your hair with a volumizing shampoo and finish with a little bit of conditioner. Don't use too much conditioner, however—you don't want the hair to be too soft.

STEP 2: To help create extra body, add a root boost or a thickening gel to towel-dried hair.

STEP 3: Dry your bangs first so that they don't dry parted or flat. Flat hair and rock star don't go well together! Once your bangs are dry, separate the rest of your hair in 1-inch sections starting at the nape of the neck and work your way up. Blow-dry section by section, starting at the nape, using a medium-size ceramic-coated round brush. Concentrate on lifting at the root for maximum body. As you get to the sections closest to the face, be sure to use a round brush to roll the sections toward the face.

STEP 4: When the hair is completely dry, begin backcombing in the crown area (the top part of your head farthest to the back, usually where your part stops). Lift the top section up and clip it out of the way and backcomb the sections underneath to build a base for height. Don't get too crazy with the backcombing, or it'll look like a bird's nest.

STEP 5: Unclip the top section of hair at the crown and place it over the backcombed hair. Smooth and blend the sections. Now is when you can get creative and do a center part or a side part—whatever you feel like.

STEP 6: Softly pull back the sides of your hair (from behind the ears) one at a time, making sure to leave a little hair over the ears. Softly secure the sides by crisscrossing two bobby pins. Feel free to use extra pins where they are needed. It doesn't matter if you can see them. Better to have too many pins than not enough. And, besides, a good rocker girlfriend always has a spare bobby pin for a friend in need.

STEP 7: Finish by using a light hair spray to lock down any fly-aways and to help maintain the style.

UP 'DO #2:
THE HIGH PONYTAIL

STEP 1: Just because you're rocking a ponytail doesn't mean you can just wash and dry your hair, pull it up, and it'll look good. It won't!

First things first: Start by using a volumizing shampoo and minimal conditioner so you get a plump pony instead of a limp one.

STEP 2: Add mousse to damp hair, then blow-dry. Don't worry too much about the blow-out being perfect. The goal here is to give the hair some volume and life. As always, dry your bangs first.

STEP 3: Once the hair is dry, throw in a shine product (I like Bumble & Bumble's Glisten drops—use sparingly!).

STEP 4: Backcomb the top of your hair to give it a little oomph.

STEP 5: You want the ponytail high on the crown to give it that bouncy rock chick look, so grab your hair from the sides and pull it up to the back of your head. Use your fingers or a comb to make sure the sides don't have hair sticking out or bunched up in any way, but be careful not to make the hair look too sleek. That's not the look we're going for here.

STEP 6: Once it's pulled back and arranged to your liking, secure the hair with a rubber band. If you want to make your pony higher and wilder, then tease the hair in the ponytail a little bit.

STEP 7: Cover the rubber hair band either with a decorative band or pull a piece of hair from the side of your pony tail and wrap it around the band, securing it with a bobby pin or by discretely tucking it under the rubber band.

STEP 8: Top off the look with a cool, rock chick–like headband (try leather, vinyl, or velvet) or scarf (try leopard print or Pucci).

VARIETY

My True Story:
Sting, Hugh Hefner, Blondes & Me

I was assigned by *Us Weekly* to cover the 2004 MusiCares Person of the Year event in Beverly Hills, honoring Sting. For whatever reason, I was seated at Hugh Hefner's table. My tablemates were Hugh, his six blonde girlfriends at the time, two of my blonde friends, and me—raven-haired and the only B cup in the group. Sting and his wife, Trudie Styler, walked by our table, and Sting looked at me and the bevy of blondes, paused for a moment, and joked, "Don't you have to be blonde to sit at this table?" Hef didn't miss a beat and responded, "Variety is the spice of life." Ah, I felt fully vindicated to be an average-height, dark-haired, nonsurgically-enhanced woman in this world. Point being: Variety IS the spice of life. Don't feel the need to conform to whatever the masses view as beautiful.

VINTAGE

By singer-songwriter Katy Perry

"I call my style "vintage trendy." I incorporate what's cool at the time with a timeless vintage piece, making the look "vintage trendy."

I love vintage pieces because they're classic and you can have them forever. But most of all, I like vintage clothing because no one else will have it and I like to wear something original. That's why I wear it, so that I'm the only one with it on.

I grew up in Santa Barbara, where swing dancing was big in the nineties. I always loved seeing the women dressed perfectly in their 1940s outfits. I have this weird body that fits into everything from the forties. I've got the boobs and butt and a really small waist, so it works for me.

I'm a huge fan of those '40s pinup girl–style onesies. They are great for summer. You just pop them on and they look hot. It's like Lolita, which is my main style influence. Then I like to pair it with some Ray Bans and accessorize with some new boots that aren't from that era.

Another way I like to mix up vintage with trendy is by wearing straight-leg pants with a vintage belt and a little bustier from the '40s along with some of those stripper-ish platform stilettos. The brands don't matter. I just put on whatever looks good. There's nothing wrong with pairing a cool vintage piece with something inexpensive and trendy from H&M, Top Shop, or even Forever 21. I do it all the time.

KATY'S MUST-HAVE VINTAGE ITEMS

1 A pencil skirt.

2 A nice pair of '70s-style leather boots. The ones that go up to your knees are great, but so are the thigh-highs.

3 Beaded, sparkly cardigan sweaters. You can wear them with any outfit.

4 Little lacy, silk vintage negligees. You can wear them to bed, or you can pair them with leggings, boots, and a little jacket, and you have an outfit.

KATY'S VINTAGE SHOPPING TIPS

■ Vintage clothing should be somewhat inexpensive.

■ Have patience and look through everything in the store.

■ It doesn't matter if the clothes look a bit worn. I wear stuff with holes in it all the time. It gives the item charm.

For a list of Anna Sui's favorite vintage stores around the world, go to page 186.

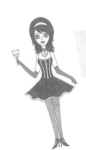

VODKA

ave Rubell, master chef, gourmet caterer, and a man who can mix a mean drink, has cooked for everyone from Nine Inch Nails to Bruce Springsteen to Madonna. He helped me create three cocktails especially for this book using black vodka (which is very rock and roll in and of itself) from England called Blavod.

The Cherry Bomb

1 shot pink lemonade

½ shot pomegranate concentrate (or 100% premium pomegranate juice)

1 shot Blavod vodka (room temperature)

1 maraschino cherry

Fill highball glass half full with crushed ice.

Pour in the pink lemonade and pomegranate juice.

Pour in the Blavod very slowly, as if you're dripping it into the glass.

Top with a maraschino cherry.

By not stirring the drink immediately, you will get the full effect of why Blavod vodka rocks. When you add in the ingredients this way (ice first, juices second, room temperature Blavod slowly dripped in on top last), you get a cool red-and-black layering effect that you don't see in other drinks. After you take a moment to appreciate the rockin' red-and-black look, feel free to stir it up and enjoy your drink.

The Party Like a Rock Star

1 shot of Original ROCKSTAR energy drink
½ shot of orange juice
1 shot Blavod vodka (room temperature)
1 green maraschino cherry

Fill highball glass half full with crushed ice.

Pour in the ROCKSTAR and orange juice.

Slowly pour in the Blavod, dripping it into the glass.

Top with a green maraschino cherry. (You can buy these at specialty beverage stores like Beverages & More.)

Before stirring, you'll see a cool orange-and-greenish layering effect. Once you stir it up, the drink takes on an even cooler muddy green color and tastes like an old-fashioned gumball.

The Black & Blue

1 shot Curacao (the blue liqueur)
1.5 shots Pellegrino sparkling water
1 shot Blavod vodka
1 blue maraschino cherry

Pour the Curacao and Pellegrino into a champagne flute.

Slowly pour the Blavod into the glass.

Top with a blue maraschino cherry.

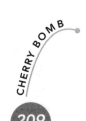

CHERRY BOMB

209

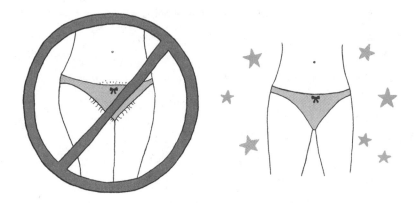

WAXING: A GUIDE

"I love Brazilians. They ought to be compulsory at 15, don't you think?"
~VICTORIA BECKHAM

"You've changed my life."
~GWYNETH PALTROW TO HER WAXER AFTER HER FIRST BRAZILIAN WAX

"It feels like a baby's butt, only all over."
~KIRSTIE ALLEY

f Gwen Stefani's husband, Gavin Rossdale, were naming his band today, it would've been called Bald instead of Bush. Okay, so maybe Gavin wasn't really thinking of a woman's nether regions when he named his alt-rock band, but it's what everyone thinks about when they hear the word *bush*, right? Well, not anymore. Nowadays, most women don't sport a bush down there. That was a cavewoman and 1970s thing. What's in now are hairless honey pots or, to use my favorite term, *glamourpussies*.

Here's the lowdown on what to do down below, but first a warning: There is no standardized list of bikini waxes. This list should give you an idea of the most popular styles and the terminology, but always talk to your waxer about what you want—in detail—first.

TYPES OF WAX STYLES

REGULAR BIKINI WAX: This is your mother's kind of waxing style. (Sorry for that visual.) You leave your undies on and they wax off whatever hair is trying to escape from your panty line.

BRAZILIAN BIKINI WAX: This is the removal of hair from (and including) your butt and anus to the entire vaginal area, including the labia, with the exception of a thin strip of hair (aka the landing strip) above the vulva. This is one of the procedures you want to discuss with your waxer in detail, because some salons consider a Brazilian to be as I just described it, while others maintain that a Brazilian means taking it all off (sometimes called the "Full Brazilian"). Bonus fact: It's called the Brazilian because it was popularized in Brazil, where the women wear very tiny G-string bikinis on the beaches and therefore need to remove more hair than one would normally have to when wearing a regular bikini.

THE PLAYBOY BIKINI WAX: Everything goes except for a very narrow, vertical strip of hair, usually two to three inches long, above your vaginal area. All of your hair is removed from the labia, butt, and anus. This is a popular look for the women who pose for *Playboy*, hence the name. Note: Some salons, such as Pink Cheeks in Sherman Oaks, California, consider waxing your panty line sides into a V shape to be a Playboy, so talk to your waxer about which version you want.

THE HOLLYWOOD, THE SPHYNX, THE BARE-ALL BIKINI WAX, THE FULL MONTY, AND THE KOJAK: These are all names for going completely hairless down there. If you don't know the references, here you go: A sphynx is a hairless cat from Egypt. *Kojak* was a popular TV show in the '70s starring a bald lead actor named Telly Savalas. *The Full Monty* was a British film featuring men stripping down to nothing. This procedure entails saying good-bye to every bit of hair from your Happy Trail down to your vagina and up and around to your buttocks. It's what Britney Spears, Paris Hilton, and Lindsay Lohan have shown off when getting out of their cars without panties on.

THUMBPRINT BIKINI WAX: A small amount of hair is left above your lovely lady parts that is about the size of a thumbprint. Everything else is waxed off.

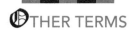

LANDING STRIP (SEE BRAZILIAN): This is a synonym for the thin vertical strip of hair that some people leave intact when they get a Brazilian wax. Some think of it as a landing strip for an airplane. To me, this just looks like a mistake. Like, "Oops. I think you missed a spot!" I say if you're going to take off that much hair, finish the job and take it all off.

HAPPY TRAIL: Like all men, some women have a thin strip of hair that travels from below their belly button to their vaginal area, jokingly called a Happy Trail because it leads a man to her goodies. If you have one, wax it off. (Britney Spears's people apparently didn't get the memo, because when she appeared on the cover of *Rolling Stone* in 1999, her Happy Trail was shockingly visible.)

DECORATIONS: The newest trend is to decorate the area in question with crystals or body gems. Sadie Frost, Elle McPherson, and Naomi Campbell are reportedly fans of this trend.

DESIGNS: This is more costly, because it takes a precise hand to wax and pluck your hair into pretty shapes like a heart, a lightning bolt, a star, your boyfriend's initials, or any other design you might request.

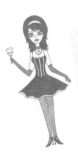

Gotha Stewart Tip: *If you have a hair emergency that requires you to shave—say, things are heating up on a date and you didn't get waxed that week—sneak into the bathroom, apply conditioner as shaving cream, and use your man's heavy-duty razor (throw out the blade afterward).*

THE NO-DUH LIST ON WAXING

■ Rock stars like hairless women.

■ The more hair you take off, the more expensive it will be.

■ Yes, it hurts. Do a shot of whiskey before you go in.

■ No, it's not embarrassing. These women have seen more kitty than Ron

CARRIE BORZILLO-VRENNA

Jeremy, Gene Simmons, and Tommy Lee combined. Nothing will surprise them. Think of your waxer the same way you think of your gynecologist.

■ Yes, oral sex is more fun if you wax. Yes, you'll be more sensitive.

■ No, you won't catch a cold because your muff warmer is gone.

Q&A WITH CYNTHIA ESSER-THORIN, OWNER OF PINK CHEEKS, WHOSE CLIENTELLE OVER THE YEARS HAS INCLUDED PAMELA AN-DERSON, PINK, SANDRA BULLOCK, JULIA ROBERTS, JANET JACKSON, MANDY MOORE, AND OTHERS.

Q: Is it true that Pamela Anderson revolutionized waxing by being the first celeb to come in and get it all taken off?
A: Yes. She came in and said, "Cindy, can you wax my lips?" And I said, "What? Your lips?" And she said, "Yes, take all of it off." I said to her, "No. That is going to hurt, sweetie." But she really wanted it, so I did it and it looked so beautiful. I said to her, "Pamela, you are really onto something here." That was in the early '90s, and we've been waxing girls like this ever since.

Q: What are your most popular waxes?
A: The full bikini is the most common. It's clean and hygienic, and with all the sexual freedom these days, it makes a woman feel confident. The Playboy Bikini runs a close second. For those who are phobic about seeming prepubescent, the Playboy leaves a nice patch of hair up top.

Q: Any advice for first timers?
A: Don't shave, cut, trim, or buzz!!! Taking Advil before you come in helps lessen the pain, psychologically. First timers should wax a few days before an event in case the hair down there is thick—sometimes the hair follicles being pulled out backward create blood spots that need to settle (this can take a day or two) and/or the client may have some ingrown hairs that we need to extract, and that takes a few days to heal up. Girls prepping for hot dates, brides, vacationers, etc. should come in three to four days before an occasion.

Q: Why do you think rock stars love it bare down there?
A: Because men aren't down there to floss their teeth! It's instantly at-tractive. And hair holds odor, so no hair means you're odorless.

VIVIENNE WESTWOOD

𝕎hat 𝕄akes 𝕍ibienne 𝕎estwood 𝕉ock?

Long before Vivienne Westwood was a line in a Gwen Stefani song, and even before she felled supermodel Naomi Campbell with her ten-inch platform shoes, Vivienne Westwood (born April 8, 1941, in Glossop, Derbyshire, England) was a punk. In fact, most credit Westwood as punk fashion's creator.

It all started in 1971, when Westwood and her partner, Malcolm McLaren (who later went on to manage the Sex Pistols, New York Dolls, and Bow Wow Wow), opened up a boutique called Let It Rock on King's Road in the Chelsea area of London. They started selling '50s-inspired clothes and old 78s. Over the years, the shop has been named Too Fast To Live/Too Young To Die, Sex, and Seditionaries. It is currently called World's End. And the fashions evolved from '50s rock and roll to punk rock pieces adorned with zippers, chains, and safety pins to S&M-inspired clothing such as her famed bondage pants and rubberwear.

Her most famous looks from her early days were the punk rock

CARRIE BORZILLO-VRENNA

fashions she put on the Sex Pistols and the New York Dolls and the pirate looks of Adam and the Ants and Bow Wow Wow.

Through the years, Westwood has revived the corset, made asymmetry and plaids must-haves, brought Victorian-era fashion ideas to modern times, taken the superhigh platform shoe from the fetish world to the runway (it was in 1993 that Naomi Campbell famously fell off of Westwood's electric blue platform shoes on a Paris catwalk), and given an edge to the power suit (remember that stunning chalk-striped suit Carrie Bradshaw wore to her meeting at *Vogue* in season four of *Sex and the City*? Westwood!). And let's not forget her wedding dresses—she designed the purple gown Dita Von Teese wore and the white gown Sarah Jessica Parker wears in *Sex and the City: The Movie.*

If that's not enough, even her offspring rocks! Westwood and McLaren's son Joseph Corre is the founder of the sexy lingerie line Agent Provocateur. Clearly, the gene that inspires people to create rocking clothes that rock stars love runs in the family.

𝔉amous Fans

Gwen Stefani
Dita Von Teese
Jerry Hall
Naomi Campbell
Sarah Jessica Parker

FUN FACT: *Gwen Stefani name-checks Vivienne Westwood in her song "Rich Girl."*

CHERRY BOMB

WORK IT

L et's face it. Only Victoria's Secret models seem to be blessed with the beauty trifecta: perfect face, hair, and body. Hardly anyone wins the genetic lottery like that. But there isn't a single female out there who doesn't have at least one great feature that they truly love. And life is all about working your best attributes and taking the attention off the ones that you don't love so much. Here's how:

Hate your butt? Play up your cleavage with a sexy, low-cut top. That will keep people's eyes up top and off your caboose.

Love your butt but hate your belly? Wear tight jeans with a voluminous top that covers your midsection but doesn't go below the top of the back pockets on your jeans.

Got skinny lips or a big nose? Move the focus onto your eyes by going for some dramatic eye makeup and extra-long and luscious lashes.

Think you're too short? Not so. You're just petite, and that means you can wear looks that tall gals can't pull off, such as short-shorts, micro-minis, Kewpie doll girlie dresses, mini-jumpers, baby-doll dresses, and extra-high heels. (To make yourself look taller, go for a monochromatic look.)

Think you're too tall? Work that length with the looks that petite girls don't rock as well: high-waisted pants, wide-legged pants, floor-length dresses, and ballet flats.

Love your legs but hate your belly? Wear a short baby-doll dress or a loose-fitting, A-line minidress.

Love your arms? Cap sleeves, puffy sleeves, sleeveless tops, and halters will look hot on you. Add a bracelet that you wear on your bicep. Hate your arms? Wear three-quarter-length sleeves.

X-RATED MOVIES

By adult film star Joanna Angel, aka The Punk Rock Princess

"I think it's good for couples to watch porn together for a few reasons. First of all, if you aren't watching porn together, well, then there's a pretty good chance that the husband is watching porn by himself and the wife doesn't know, which means there's a secret in the relationship. It's always good for two people who are sharing a life to have things out in the open. I don't think anyone in a relationship should be doing anything on a regular basis without the other person knowing. It's just a very bad foundation. Also, sometimes when a couple has been together for a long time they can run out of ideas for things to do with each other in the bedroom, and porn can definitely be inspiring.

CARRIE BORZILLO-VRENNA

218

YOHJI YAMAMOTO

What Makes Yohji Yamamoto Rock?

Japanese designers are popular with the rock and roll set, and Yohji Yamamoto is at the top of the list. Gwen Stefani name-checked him in her ode to Japanese style in "Harajuku Girls." Evanescence's Amy Lee is a fan, and so is Alanis Morissette. British rockers Placebo have worn the Y-3 sneakers he created with Adidas on tour. Even fellow designers sing his praises—Giorgio Armani has called Yamamoto's work "poetic."

Considered one of the most influential and important designers today, Yamamoto (born October 3, 1943, in Yokohama, Japan) is known for his rebellious designs, which often veer extremely left of that season's trends. His signature style is loose, oversized clothes in head-to-toe black. Instead of celebrating the female form with figure-hugging designs, the avant-garde designer opts to conceal her in a cloak of mystery. This makes him a fantastic designer among larger ladies or women who don't want to show off all of their goodies.

And what makes this sometimes strange but always fascinating designer really rock is that, well, he *really rocks*. He's played guitar in and fronted his own rock band.

CHERRY BOMB

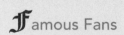

Famous Fans

Gwen Stefani
Amy Lee
Alicia Keys
Mary J. Blige
Ali Larter
Alanis Morissette

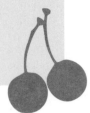

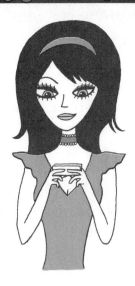

ZIG-ZAGS

𝕿𝖍𝖊 𝕮𝖔𝖔𝖑 𝖂𝖆𝖞 𝖙𝖔 𝕽𝖔𝖑𝖑 𝖆 𝕵𝖔𝖎𝖓𝖙

𝕿ools

1 ¼ Zig-Zag rolling papers
1 small pair of scissors
Some weed

DIRECTIONS

STEP 1: Break up the bud with a pair of scissors until it's light and fluffy, discarding the stems, leaves, and seeds, if any. (Good pot shouldn't have seeds.) Note: Scissors trump fingers because resin sticks to your skin and you want to keep that resin in the bud to enjoy. And, besides, taking scissors to a fat bud is like manicuring a bonsai tree, and that's fun!

STEP 2: Make a ¼-inch fold on the bottom half of the rolling paper. (The sticky side should be up and facing you.)

CHERRY BOMB

STEP 3: Pack the middle crease of the folded rolling paper with as much light and fluffy bud as you can fit in there. You want to pack it in nice and tight and distribute it evenly from left to right.

STEP 4: This is the tricky part. Pick up the open joint with your left pointer finger and middle finger, as if you're making a peace sign, and then turn it on its side, moving the pointer finger closer to you, making a sideways scissor-kick formation. Put your right pointer finger and middle finger in the same position. You should be holding onto the joint with your two pointer fingers in front of the paper, the tips of those fingers touching. Likewise, your two middle fingers should be behind the paper, and those tips should be touching. Next, for balance and rolling reasons, your two thumbs should be hanging out below your pointers and—you guessed it—your thumb tips should be touching.

STEP 5: If you placed your fingers in the right position, you should now be able to roll the joint with your thumbs by rolling and tucking the paper upward (away from you). Take your time manipulating the joint with this rolling-upward movement of your thumbs until the joint is even and tight.

STEP 6: Lick the glue side of the paper (it should be facing inward toward you). Real pros then put the entire joint in their mouths and gently suck on it until it's nice and tight.

STEP 7: Trim the ends with scissors. You don't want two tightly twisted joint ends. You want them slightly opened.

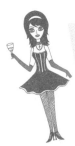

Gotha Stewart Tip: *Don't roll the joint too tight, and don't pinch the ends of either side too tight either; it'll be hard to draw the air you need.*

EPILOGUE

Which Rock Chick Are You Most Like?

1 The outfit you're most comfortable in is . . .

a. a tight pair of jeans, a T-shirt, and a leather jacket.

b. a high-fashion dress, oversized sunglasses, and funky accessories.

c. Dickies Girl pants, a hoodie, and sneakers.

d. a vintage party dress, sneakers, and heavy eyeliner.

e. skinny jeans, a bra, and REALLY heavy eyeliner.

2 The kind of guys who make your heart skip a beat are . . .

a. athletes, actors, and songwriters.

b. singers, bassists, and guitarists.

c. skater boys and punks.

d. British boys and electronic musicians.

e. British boys and bad boys.

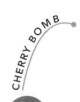

3 On a sunny summer afternoon, you like to . . .

    a. soak up the sun.

    b. shade yourself from the sun.

    c. kick the sun's ass for shining too brightly!

    d. talk smack about the sun.

    e. sleep in.

4 Your favorite female singers are . . .

    a. Janis Joplin, Melissa Etheridge, and Loretta Lynn.

    b. Blondie's Debbie Harry, Madonna, Missing Persons' Dale Bozzio.

    c. Alanis Morissette, the Distillers' Brody Dalle, Courtney Love.

    d. None. You like the boys better.

    e. Billie Holiday, Etta James, Macy Gray.

5 Your favorite hairdo is . . .

    a. long, wavy, and natural.

    b. retro chic, blond, and always "done."

    c. spiced up with a streak of pink.

    d. long and '60s-ish.

    e. a beehive.

6 A mean girl gets in your face and says something nasty to you. How do you handle it?

    a. You laugh it off and move on.

    b. You're too intimidating for anyone to get that close to you.

    c. You spit at her and flip the double bird.

    d. You lash out at her on MySpace or in a song.

    e. You scream at her and get into a catfight.

7 Your favorite workout is . . .

   a. surfing.

   b. running.

   c. tramping.

   d. hypnotherapy.

   e. nothing.

8 One of your favorite accessories is . . .

   a. a leather jacket.

   b. a houndstooth scarf.

   c. a black studded belt.

   d. vintage earrings.

   e. a new tattoo.

9 You could be deemed . . .

   a. an All-American Girl.

   b. a Harajuku Girl.

   c. a Dickies Girl.

   d. a Retro Girl.

   e. a Troubled Girl.

10 Which best describes you?

   a. You like a good beer buzz early in the morning.

   b. You were born to blossom but bloomed to perish.

   c. You think you're the motherfucking princess.

   d. Someone messed up your mental health.

   e. You've been black, but you've come back. Yes, yes, yes.

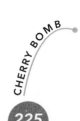

CHERRY BOMB

IF YOU ANSWERED . . .	THEN YOU ARE MOST LIKE . . .
Mostly As . . .	Sheryl Crow
Mostly Bs . . .	Gwen Stefani
Mostly Cs . . .	Avril Lavigne
Mostly Ds . . .	Lily Allen
Mostly Es . . .	Amy Winehouse

ACKNOWLEDGMENTS

A COLOSSAL THANK-YOU TO . . .

My husband, Chris Vrenna, for making life exciting, my first pair of Vivienne Westwood heels, his stellar research skills, and invaluable help from brainstorming title ideas to pulling all-nighters to finish the book.

My dad for turning me onto the Rolling Stones at age seven, my sister for covering for me when I snuck out to go see my first rock concert at age fourteen, my mom for not flipping out when I brought my first musician boyfriend home at age sixteen, and the rest of my family for their love and support.

My "Rock Chick Focus Group" for taste-testing my absinthe collection, sitting pretty for the smoky eye demonstration, jumping on my trampoline, and/or test-driving my quizzes: Tina Patrick, Jennifer Kashdan, Wendy Ellis, Mollie Johnson, Patty Micciche, Dana Stangel, Rhonda J. Wilson, and Alexandra Greenberg of MSO PR, who also helped with publicity for the book.

My contributors for taking the time to share their rockin' advice and tips: Tori Amos, Joanna Angel, Dean Banowetz, Cheryl Burke, Dr. Ava Cadell, Cherie Currie, Cynthia Esser-Thorin, Cynthia Freund,

Imogen Heap, Jessicka, Betsey Johnson, Christian Joy, NicoleLee Suicide, Lisa Loeb, Mezghan, Samantha Maloney, Terri Nunn, Tera Patrick, Katy Perry, Louise Post, Nicole Powers, Dave Rubell, Anna Sui, Viper Room's Melissa Renee Hernandez and Anna Geyer, Kat Von D., and Dita Von Teese.

My agent, Holly Root at Waxman Literary Agency, for taking ten ideas and helping me come up with one insanely fun book to write and talking me off the ledge when necessary.

My editor, Emily Westlake, for totally "getting it" and for being the coolest editor a girl could ever hope for. And everyone else at Simon Spotlight Entertainment, including Jennifer Bergstrom and Michael Broussard for their support and for making it happen, Yaffa Jaskoll for the most amazing cover, and Jaime Putorti for a rockin' interior. You all rock!

My illustrator, Liz Adams, for making the book come to life. I'm honored to have a rock chick like you be a part of this book.

My photo shoot team for making me look my best: Piper Ferguson, Apollo Staar, Dina Amsden, Memosa Meadow, Allison Nichole, and Lelah Foster; and Amy Liu of Miss Sixty for the rockin' clothes.

All my other friends or colleagues who offered up leads, ideas, help, advice, and/or support in one important way or another: Erin Culley, Marc Spitz, Lonn Friend, Jeannie Long, Erik Stein, Kevin Raub, William Berrol, Jim Dinda, Marisa Laudadio, Ken Phillips, Daniel House and rockandrolldating.com, Roxanne Rubell, Wendy and Alan Sartirana, Deb Jhaj, Michael Grgas, Wen Chang, Priscilla, Sherrie Toews, the songwriters and music publishers who allowed me to use their lyrics, and all of my MySpace friends (www.myspace.com/carrieborzillo vrenna) who regularly chimed in on titles, photos, and song lists, and who cheered me along.

ABOUT THE AUTHOR

Carrie Borzillo-Vrenna has been covering the music/entertainment industry for sixteen years. She has written about music for *Billboard*, *Spin*, RollingStone.com, and *Alternative Press*; about celebrities for *People*, *Us Weekly*, and *Teen People*; and dished out sex/relationship advice for *Gene Simmons Tongue*. Her first book, *Eyewitness Nirvana: The Day by Day Chronicles*, received rave reviews. She lives in Los Angeles with her Grammy award–winning husband, Chris Vrenna (Marilyn Manson, Gnarls Barkley). Visit www.carriebv.com.

PHOTO CREDITS

Photographer: Piper Ferguson, www.piperferguson.com
Photography Team: Apollo Staar (assistant), Lelah Foster (intern)
Stylist: Dina Amsden
Makeup: Memosa Meadow
Hair: Allison Nichole

LYRICS PERMISSIONS

"Cherry Bomb" by Kim Fowley and Joan Larkin
    © 1976 by Peermusic Ltd. (and as designated by copublisher)
    Used by permission. All rights reserved.
"Ur So Gay" lyrics courtesy of Katy Perry and When I'm Rich You'll Be
    My Bitch/Warner-Chappell Publishing (ASCAP)
    Used by permission.
"Bad Reputation" lyrics courtesy of Jett Pack Music Inc./Lagunatic
    Music & Filmworks, Inc. Written by Joan Jett, Kenny Laguna,
    Ritchie Cordell, and Martin Kupersmith.
    Used by permission.
"Fake Friends" lyrics courtesy of Jett Pack Music Inc./Lagunatic Music
    & Filmworks, Inc. Written by Joan Jett and Kenny Laguna.
    Used by permission.
"Sex (I'm A . . .)" lyrics courtesy of Berlin Era Music/Xytyryan Rex
    Music/Malladin Music BMI. Written by John Crawford, David Dia-
    mond, and Terri Nunn. Used by permission.